'As with any chronic disease we rarely have the opportunity to cure, but we do have the opportunity to treat the patient with respect. Such an experience may be the greatest gift a doctor can give an obese patient.'

(From Stunkard A. Talking with patients. In: Stunkard A, Wadden T, editors. *Obesity: Theory and Therapy*. New York: Raven Press; 1993)

Weight Management

Weight Management

A Practitioner's Guide

Dympna Pearson RD
Consultant Dietitian and Trainer, Leicester

Clare Grace RD, PhD
*Obesity Specialist Dietitian, King's College Hospital NHS
Foundation Trust, London*

WILEY-BLACKWELL

A John Wiley & Sons, Ltd., Publication

This edition first published 2012
© 2012 by Dympna Pearson and Clare Grace

Wiley-Blackwell is an imprint of John Wiley & Sons, formed by the merger of Wiley's global Scientific, Technical and Medical business with Blackwell Publishing.

Registered Office
John Wiley & Sons, Ltd, The Atrium, Southern Gate, Chichester, West Sussex, PO19 8SQ, UK

Editorial Offices
9600 Garsington Road, Oxford, OX4 2DQ, UK
The Atrium, Southern Gate, Chichester, West Sussex, PO19 8SQ, UK
2121 State Avenue, Ames, Iowa 50014-8300, USA

For details of our global editorial offices, for customer services and for information about how to apply for permission to reuse the copyright material in this book please see our website at www.wiley.com/wiley-blackwell.

Library of Congress Cataloging-in-Publication Data

Pearson, Dympna.
Weight management : a practitioner's guide / Dympna Pearson, Clare Grace.
   p.   cm.
  Includes bibliographical references and index.
  ISBN 978-1-4051-8559-2 (pbk.)
 1. Obesity–Treatment.   2. Reducing diets.   3. Exercise therapy.   I. Grace, Clare.   II. Title.
  RC628.P36 2012
  616.3′98–dc23

2012007651

A catalogue record for this book is available from the British Library.

Wiley also publishes its books in a variety of electronic formats. Some content that appears in print may not be available in electronic books.

Cover Image: Mark Wragg/iStockphoto
Cover design by Steve Thompson

Set in 10/12.5pt Sabon by SPi Publisher Services, Pondicherry, India
Printed and bound in Malaysia by Vivar Printing Sdn Bhd

1   2012

Contents

Foreword

With one in four adults in England now obese, and almost a third of children being either overweight or obese, it is easy to see why obesity is one of the most serious and complex health challenges we are facing in the UK today. The financial cost to the NHS, according to current estimates, is more than £4 billion, and yet obesity is a health issue that, paradoxically, attracts enormous public interest but still remains a worryingly low priority within medicine.

The costs to patient health are well documented, and we know that obesity is a contributing factor in cardiovascular disease, type 2 diabetes, cancer and early death. But beyond that, the social and psychological cost to people with obesity can be enormous.

On a daily basis we are confronted with stories in the media telling us how fat we are becoming, and of the latest faddy diet, obesity 'miracle pill' or 'undeserving, greedy over-eaters' receiving NHS-funded gastric band operations.

With this continued negative focus, it is unsurprising that the perception remains that dealing with obesity is as simple as 'eat less and do more', when all evidence suggests that there is a multitude of behavioural, environmental and genetic factors that are responsible and that, most importantly, there is no magic bullet to 'cure' obesity.

Weight Management: A Practitioner's Guide is an excellent resource which identifies the various ways practitioners can help their obese patients take control of their own weight, while challenging them to confront their own perceptions of obese patients, and make changes to their practice accordingly.

Patients with obesity do not want to be defined by their weight, and the tools, guidance and resources within this book will help practitioners help place their patients at the centre of their own care from the very first consultation, allowing them to make effective changes that will improve their health and quality of life.

Dr Clare Gerada
Chair of the Royal College of General Practitioners

Acknowledgements

We wish to express our sincere thanks to the many colleagues who have helped us with this book, in particular Karen Allen, Cheryl Flanagan, Joanne Jones and Alison Macleod for their dietetic expertise and wisdom in reviewing early versions and their ongoing enthusiasm for its development. We would like to express our gratitude to Jill McMullan and Hannah Stewart for their help with analysing the food diaries.

Also, we wish to thank our families for their love, support, encouragement and endless patience.

Introduction

The aim of this book is to support and inspire practitioners working in weight management on how best to manage obesity, with a primary focus on lifestyle interventions in adults.

There are numerous obesity textbooks guiding us on the alarming rise in the prevalence, the causes and the consequences of obesity, and the theory and evidence on how it should be managed. However, surprisingly little detailed attention has been given to the specifics of clinical practice. What is the best way of raising the issue of overweight? When and how should we assess eating and activity behaviour? What is the most effective dietary treatment? These are just some of the many issues that arise when working with overweight patients, and which this book aims to address.

It brings together evidence of best practice, considers in detail the practical application of these approaches and provides clear answers to frequently encountered challenges. It is packed with practical tools and examples from practice and will guide you step by step through a framework of care for overweight and obese individuals.

Although we now know more about what works in weight management, the complexity and relapsing nature of obesity highlights the importance of further investment in training and research. Many health professionals report low confidence in their abilities to help obese patients and this is likely to have a negative impact on treatment outcomes, as well as the patient's and the practitioner's experience. Practitioners often relate poor confidence to inadequate training in the practical lifestyle recommendations and behavioural approaches to weight management. While this book is not a substitute for high-quality skills training, it does provide an opportunity for practitioners to learn through self-reflection, gather additional knowledge and insight, and relate their experiences to those presented in practical examples. The book is also designed to allow practitioners to dip into relevant sections as the need or the practice-related question arises.

Much of the recent focus in obesity management has centred on prevention of overweight, particularly in children. This includes pre-conception and maternal nutrition, weaning and infant feeding, as well as pre-school nutrition. These interventions early in life are inextricably linked to the whole family, making it impossible to separate management of obesity from prevention. It is essential that sufficient focus is given to treatment of adults with established obesity, as their behaviours will be modelled within families and by children.

This book focuses on lifestyle treatment in adults, primarily one-to-one interventions, and does not address the complexities of childhood obesity, which merits its own dedicated practitioner guide.

The first section begins by exploring why treating obesity is so important and considers some of the key causal issues involved. It then explores practitioners' attitudes to obesity and how these might influence practice. This is followed by a brief overview of the evidence for lifestyle treatments, with additional information on drug and surgical interventions as adjuncts to lifestyle programmes. The second section guides the reader through the practical aspects of a patient-centred weight-management intervention and includes suggestions on how to adhere to best practice when time is limited. The ongoing challenge of weight maintenance and how to evaluate the impact of treatment are also addressed. Given obesity management is littered with myths and misconceptions, these are the subject of the final chapter, and practical examples are provided to help the practitioner relate this information to their daily practice.

We hope you find this book helpful.

Note to readers

Throughout this book we have chosen to use the term 'patient' rather than 'client'. This reflects our belief that obesity is a chronic disease, and individuals often need support to manage, not only their weight, but also the associated diseases. We recognise that some readers may prefer to substitute the term 'client', particularly if working in non-health care settings.

1 Background Information

1 Why Treat Obesity?

'Obesity poses a threat on a similar scale to climate change' [1]

What is the scale of the obesity problem?

Obesity is one of the most serious and complex health challenges faced by the UK, Europe and most of the rest of the world. There has been a dramatic doubling in its prevalence over the last 25 years with most adults in England now overweight, and 1 in 4 obese (24% men; 25% women) [2]. Alarmingly similar trends have been observed in children, with 14.4% of 2–10 year olds obese in 2009 [3]. If current trends continue, future prevalence predictions are dire, with suggestions that 9 in 10 adults in England could be obese by 2050 [4].

This will have profound cost implications for the NHS and the wider economy. Current estimates for the NHS suggest obesity costs £4.2 billion/year, with wider economic costs (reduced productivity, loss of earnings, increased benefits) of £16 billion/year. If future prevalence predictions are accurate, this may rise to £10 billion/year and £50 billion/year, respectively [4].

A strong social inequality exists in the prevalence of obesity, although the factors responsible are unclear: in men, 18% are obese in social class I versus 28% in social class V; in women, 10% are obese in social class I versus 25% in social class V [5]. Unfortunately, there is limited information on whether prevalence varies by ethnicity as most surveys only include small numbers from various ethnic groups. However, in 2004, a higher prevalence of obesity was found in black African, black Caribbean and Pakistani women compared to the general population [6].

Why does it matter?

Obesity is known to shorten life, is a risk factor for a range of major co-morbidities and can have profound effects on an individual's psychological and social well being. There are also wider economic and social consequences for society that make addressing obesity a compelling, albeit challenging, issue.

Weight Management: A Practitioner's Guide, First Edition. Dympna Pearson and Clare Grace.
© 2012 Dympna Pearson and Clare Grace. Published 2012 by Blackwell Publishing Ltd.

Obesity and early death

Obesity shortens life

Up to 13 years of life can be lost in obese men and up to 8 years in obese women [7]

Obesity increases the risk of dying early, particularly in men. In young adults there is a 50% greater risk of early death in those with body mass index (BMI) above 30 kg/m^2 compared to healthy-weight individuals [8]. Over the years there has been debate on the precise relationship between mortality risk and obesity. However, after appropriate adjustment for confounders, an elevated BMI is clearly linked with increased risk of premature death [9–11]. Obese white men aged 20–30 years with a BMI greater than 45 kg/m^2 are likely to lose 13 years of their life and for women with similar characteristics this can be up to 8 years [7]. The link between mortality risk and BMI is greatest up to the age of 50 but does continue through to old age [12]. Risk can be moderated depending on the level of physical fitness, with suggestions that being overweight and inactive may account for up to 31% of early all-cause mortality [13].

Obesity and type 2 diabetes

Diabetes risk

Rapid rise above BMI 25 kg/m^2
Longer obesity duration = greater diabetes risk
Even small increases in weight increase risk

Of all the associated co-morbidities, type 2 diabetes is the most strongly linked. Increasing fat mass, particularly abdominal/visceral obesity, is well recognised as a risk factor for the development of type 2 diabetes, due to its contribution to insulin resistance and beta cell dysfunction. The BMI above which diabetes risk begins to rise rapidly is surprising low, with a 3.6-fold greater risk in women with a BMI of 23–24 kg/m^2 compared to those with a BMI <22 kg/m^2, highlighting that this association is not the sole reserve of the severely obese [14]. For those aged 40–49 years with BMI >35 kg/m^2, risk of developing diabetes has been found to be almost 80 times higher than in those with a BMI of <22 kg/m^2 [15].

The longer the duration of obesity and weight gain, the higher the level of risk, with a 3-fold elevated risk in those who have been overweight for less than 5 years versus a 5-fold risk in those who have been overweight for more than 5 years [16]. Several studies have shown that individuals with small weight gains in early adulthood of ~5–8 kg have twice the risk of diabetes compared to those who have minimised weight gain [15,17], emphasising the importance of preventing weight gain.

The risk of diabetes varies by ethnicity and is especially high in those of Asian origin. For each 5 kg weight gain, the risk of diabetes increased by 37% in whites, 38% in blacks but 84% in Asians.

Weight gain of 5 kg increases diabetes risk by 84% in Asians versus 37% in whites

Obesity and cancer

A BMI of ≥40 kg/m^2 has been associated with a 50–60% increased chance of developing cancer compared to healthy-weight individuals [9]. Obesity has been specifically implicated in cancer of the colon, endometrium and breast. A 1.5-fold greater risk of developing colorectal cancer has been found in women with a BMI greater than 29 kg/m^2 and in men with abdominal obesity (waist–hip ratio, WHR ≥ 0.99) [18,19]. Dietary factors (red and processed meats may exacerbate, while fibre and n-3 PUFA may protect) and physical inactivity (high activity levels may protect) have also been linked to the risk of colon cancer.

Obesity and cardiovascular disease

Obesity is a major modifiable risk factor for coronary heart disease. Its association with various atherogenic lipid and lipoprotein abnormalities is well recognised, including elevated total cholesterol and triglyceride, and lowered high-density lipoprotein cholesterol [20]. It is this link with atherogenesis, together with its negative impact on other coronary risk factors (hypertension, type 2 diabetes), that explains the strong positive association between the incidence of coronary heart disease and obesity [21]. It has been estimated that as much as 70% of the coronary heart disease in obese women is attributable to overweight [22]. The distribution of adipose tissue is also known to be important, with central obesity increasing metabolic risk via a greater predisposition to dyslipidemia [23].

Quality of life

Research clearly illustrates that obesity has an adverse effect on health-related quality of life, with the magnitude of impairment increasing with increasing severity of obesity [24]. Conversely, improvements are reported after weight loss, although most research has explored changes after surgery rather than changes related to lifestyle approaches [25]. Obesity affects many aspects of physical and social functioning, sexual function and satisfaction, public distress and the ability to engage fully in the workplace.

Whether obesity leads to or is a consequence of depression has been hotly debated and there is a need for greater understanding of this complex relationship. A recent meta-analysis concluded that depression and obesity were reciprocal, with an increased risk of depression in the obese, and with depression being predictive for obesity [26].

Factors that increase the risk of obesity

Smoking cessation

Giving up smoking is commonly associated with an average weight gain of 7 kg [27], although this varies by age, lifestyle behaviours and socioeconomic status. There are a number of possible reasons for this link, including: the removal of the appetite suppressing effect of nicotine; an improved sense of taste and smell leading to altered food preferences; swapping oral gratification from smoking to food; and behaviourally using food in the same way as cigarettes – for example, to deal with stress, boredom, self-rewards or as a means of socialising.

Although over 80% of those quitting smoking will gain weight, the health benefits of smoking cessation far outweigh the health risks of gaining weight.

> To reach the same health risk as smoking one packet of cigarettes a day, the average smoker would need to be 55 kg overweight

As the evidence currently stands, the optimal timing of weight management and quit attempts is unclear. There is some concern that trying to control weight through lifestyle interventions while trying to quit smoking may negatively impact on the success of smoking cessation. Until it is clear that concurrent weight management does not lead to an increase in quit failure it may be wise to reserve weight-management interventions until smoking cessation has been successfully completed. However, there may be instances when an individual is so concerned about the possibility of weight gain that it adversely affects their motivation to stop smoking. Such situations require clinical judgment to determine whether individualised weight management alongside smoking cessation would be beneficial.

The provision of general advice 'to avoid gaining weight' while trying to quit smoking is generally ineffective and may hinder smoking cessation attempts. However, individualised weight-management interventions limit the extent of weight gain during the smoking cessation period, although the effect is small. The use of cognitive behavioural therapy and very low-calorie diets alongside smoking cessation treatments may be beneficial in reducing post-cessation weight gain. Longer-term studies are required and it is recommended that these strategies are reserved for use in research settings [27].

The role of physical activity in managing weight during and after smoking cessation is a little unclear, although it may be important for improved weight control over the longer term [27,28].

> Just advising people planning to stop smoking to avoid gaining weight is unhelpful and may prevent the attempt to quit.
>
> There is insufficient evidence to determine the optimal timing of weight-management interventions and smoking cessation.
>
> It may be most prudent to wait until after a successful quit attempt has been completed before considering weight-management interventions.
>
> The decision to offer individualised weight-management interventions concurrently with a quit attempt should be made on an individual basis using clinical judgment.

Certain medications

There are certain medications known to increase the risk of weight gain and some of those listed below have been associated with up to a 10 kg gain over 12 weeks [29]. It may be helpful to discuss weight-management options in instances where the prescribing of such medications is necessary and an alternative is not suitable.

- atypical antipsychotics, including clozapine;
- beta adrenergic blockers, particularly propranolol;
- insulin, when used in the treatment of type 2 diabetes mellitus;
- lithium;
- sodium valproate;
- sulphonylureas, including chlorpropamide, glibenclamide, glimepiride and glipizide;
- thiazolidinediones, including pioglitazone;
- tricyclic antidepressants, including amitriptyline.

To date there is no evidence to suggest a link between oral combined contraceptives or hormone replacement therapy and weight gain [30].

Obesity and its causes

Obesity is commonly misconstrued as a self-inflicted condition, the causes of which are simple: eating too much and exercising too little. This is far removed from the complex nature of obesity revealed by science, and such misunderstandings tend to fuel weight-related stigma and do little to enhance obesity treatments.

Why do practitioners need a good understanding of obesity causes?

Developing a broad understanding of the complex biological and environmental factors involved in the development of obesity may have a number of important benefits:

1 **Positive impact on the practitioner's attitudes to obese people (Chapter 2)** Acknowledging obesity is not self-inflicted, and patients are often pushing back against strong biological tendencies and a challenging environment helps practitioners understand the challenge of weight management.
2 **Improvement of the assessment process** A better understanding of the factors involved in obesity development may lead to a more sophisticated assessment of these elements.
3 **Improvement of the therapeutic relationship** Discussing issues of predisposition can convey understanding and optimism. The information that some people are more predisposed to obesity can be helpful for those who find it difficult to understand, and accept, why they find it harder to control their weight than others. It may allay feelings of self-blame, guilt and shame and is likely to convey a sense of support and understanding on the part of the practitioner.

Society views obesity as the result of personal failure (often lack of willpower) rather than influenced by environmental and genetic factors. Patients (and some health professionals) often view obesity in the same way. Summarising for patients what science tells us about the causes of obesity can counter these misconceptions, may allay guilt and self-blame, and can empower patients to address their obesity.

Consider this

If, as an obese person, a patient's starting point for managing their weight is this:
'I'm failing to lose weight because I don't have enough willpower. Why am I so useless at dieting when lots of my friends seem to have no difficulty? I know it's my fault and I need to do something about it but I don't know where to start. I suppose I just need to try harder but I'm not sure I can.'
Ask yourself:

1 What is the likely effect of their beliefs about the causes of their obesity on their self-esteem?
2 How confident are they likely to be about their ability to change behaviour and weight?
3 Is this a good place from which to begin a weight-management programme?

After discussion, the patient's attitude could be this:
'I've struggled with my weight for years and I've always blamed myself. Why couldn't I just eat less and do more exercise? It sounds so simple but I've failed at it time and time again. Now I understand that although some of it is clearly about me and the choices I make, it's not all my fault. That makes me feel so much better about myself and when I feel better about myself I eat less. Knowing that some people's bodies are much better set up to control weight is really helpful. I know my weight is always going to be something I need to take real care with, but I feel determined now to do something about this.'

What are the causes of obesity?

There is no single cause of obesity and no one dominant causal factor. Rather, obesity develops as a consequence of a complex mix of genetic and environmental factors, the contributions and relevancies of which vary from one individual to another. This degree of causal complexity is elegantly illustrated in the Foresight Report: (http://www.bis.gov.uk/assets/bispartners/foresight/docs/obesity/obesity_final_part2.pdf) (see diagram on page 84).

At the most simplistic level, energy balance explains why weight gain occurs. If energy consumed from food/drink exceeds that expended through physical activity (and metabolism), a positive energy balance occurs and weight gain is the result. However, this explanatory model provides an incomplete picture and does not highlight the many complicated mechanisms that influence why someone might consume more energy, or do little physical activity.

It is now widely accepted that the rapid rise in the prevalence of obesity has been driven by technological advances which have dramatically changed the way we live. This has impacted on work patterns, modes of transport, food production, meal preparation and shopping practices, and this changed environment has revealed an underlying tendency for many people to gain weight. The Foresight report [1] describes this as 'passive obesity': an almost involuntary process of weight gain where the environmental drivers of obesity have been so overwhelming that weight gain is inevitable for many people. This highlights the inaccuracy of considering obesity a self-inflicted condition in which sole responsibility for change lies with the individual.

At an individual level the causes of obesity are numerous and will vary from person to person. Across an individual's life span the causes of weight gain may also change. This underlines the importance of comprehensive assessment (Chapter 6) so that the specific factors that have contributed to weight gain over time can be identified, and modifiable elements addressed through management.

Biology and genes

Food intake and appetite regulation

Substantial advances have occurred in our understanding of the specific mechanisms involved in appetite regulation, many of which have come from animal models of obesity. The body attempts to regulate weight and food intake through a complex biological system of hormonal and neural pathways and feedback loops. Appetite regulation is extremely complex and centres on the hypothalamus and brain stem as the key regulators of energy balance in the brain. They receive information from the gastrointestinal tract, adipose tissue and circulation about current fat stores and nutritional status, and analyse and then modify responses accordingly. There are numerous complex pathways and signals involved and much has been learnt about signals and systems that stimulate (Neuropeptide Y, Agouti protein, melanin concentrating hormone) or terminate (POMC, corticotrophin-releasing factor) feeding. Leptin, secreted by adipose tissue, is probably the best-known signal and seems to function as a trigger to increase feeding when fat stores are low. Leptin levels fall as fat stores decline, leading to an increase in hunger and food-seeking behaviour. Conversely, as fat stores increase higher leptin levels signal the hypothalamus, satiety occurs, food intake subsequently falls and equilibrium is achieved. However, there is a great deal still to be learnt about the functioning of this complex system and the interactions between the many signals and pathways.

As the obesity epidemic illustrates, this control system has struggled to adapt to our rapidly changing environment and 'the pace of technological progress has outstripped human evolution' [1]. It seems that appetite regulation may be more tightly controlled in naturally thin people, with greater precision in the matching between energy consumed and energy expended. In those predisposed to obesity, the appetite control system may be less proficient at matching, and unless eating and activity behaviours are consciously controlled, weight gain occurs. Research has illustrated that, appetite control mechanisms can be easily overridden by the sight, smell, palatability and availability of foods [31] – sensory factors that are so abundant in today's environment.

Energy expenditure

Research has explored the 'energy sparing' aspects of metabolism to determine whether there might be components of energy expenditure which make substantial contributions to the aetiology of obesity. There is no evidence to support the idea that obesity is caused by a slow metabolism. Indeed, research suggests that resting energy expenditure tends to be higher in obese people because of the higher metabolic cost of larger body sizes. After adjustment for body weight and composition there is hardly any difference between resting metabolism in obese and lean people [32]. Indeed, no physiological differences have been found that might explain why lean people avoid weight gain in the current environment, and in studies where overfeeding has occurred similar rates of weight gain or loss have been seen.

Early growth patterns

Nutrition and growth in the womb and early childhood seem to influence obesity risk in later life, although the mechanisms for this are unclear. Low-birth-weight babies have a higher risk of heart disease and diabetes in adulthood, and this may be linked with rapid weight gain and feeding practices in the first few months of life [33]. Metabolism may be plastic in the first few months of life and the nutritional environment may play a role in 'setting' the baby's metabolic pathway. This highlights the importance of healthy nutrition and lifestyle choices in early life.

Eating and activity behaviours

These are clearly critical elements of influence on obesity; however, attempts to understand their precise contribution are hampered by the methods available to measure food intake and physical activity. Measuring dietary intake relies on reported rather than actual intake and obesity is known to be associated with substantial under-reporting of energy intake. Nonetheless, a number of dietary risk factors have been identified, including high-energy dense foods, diets high in fat and low in fibre, sugary drinks and large portion sizes.

The obesogenic environment

Recent environmental changes are commonly linked with the increasing prevalence of obesity, although the magnitude of their involvement isn't fully understood. Technological advances (cars, washing machines, dishwashers) have reduced the effort required for many everyday activities and together with reduced occupational activity are likely to encourage obesity. Likewise the increased access and availability of relatively cheap, but not necessarily healthy food, and increasingly unstructured meal patterns make the healthy choice more challenging.

Health benefits of modest weight loss

Although many patients will strive to achieve an 'ideal' body weight, the inherent challenges in weight management may mean this isn't feasible (depending on baseline BMI) with dietary intervention alone. In fact, it may not be necessary. There is good evidence to support the value of modest weight loss in improving health and psychological well being. Indeed, it can be argued that losing and sustaining modest amounts of weight is better than losing and then regaining substantial quantities of weight.

It is recommended that weight-loss targets are not based simply on weight alone but include the patient's existing co-morbidities and risks. In those with a BMI between 25 and 35 kg/m², where co-morbidities are less likely, a 5–10% weight loss is often sufficient to reduce cardiovascular and metabolic risk. However, in those with a BMI greater than 35 kg/m², where co-morbidities may be present, weight loss of 15–20% may be necessary before sustained improvements to co-morbidities occur [29].

BMI 25–35 kg/m²	5–10% target weight loss
BMI >35 kg/m²	15–20% target weight loss

Modest sustained weight loss (5–10%) has been associated with the following:

- **Mortality**   Reduced all-cause mortality in those with diabetes and lower cancer- and diabetes-related mortality in obese women with some obesity-related co-morbidity [34].
- **Asthma**   Improved lung function (if more than 10 kg lost) [35].
- **Arthritis**   Reduced osteoarthritis-related disability (5% weight loss associated with improved function and reduced pain) [36]. Improved mobility and reduced pain reported in adults over 60 years with established osteoarthritis [37].
- **Blood pressure**   A reduction of 3.8–4.4 mm Hg in systolic and 3–3.6 mm Hg in diastolic blood pressure at 12 months with a 5 kg loss, and a 6 mm Hg fall in systolic and 4.6 mm Hg in diastolic blood pressure at 2 years with a 10 kg loss [38,39].
- **Diabetes**   In those with impaired glucose tolerance, lifestyle treatments and modest weight loss can prevent or delay the onset of type 2 diabetes (58% reduction in diabetes incidence) [40]. In obese patients with type 2 diabetes, a 5 kg loss has been found to reduce HbA1c by 0.28% at 12 months [34,39].
- **Lipid profile**   Modest weight loss is associated with reductions in low-density lipoprotein, total cholesterol and triglycerides and with increased levels of high-density lipoprotein [34,41].

Conclusion

If current predictions are correct, in 40 years' time the majority of UK adults will be obese. This will have overwhelming cost implications for health care and the wider economy. Given the profound effect of obesity on morbidity and mortality and the substantial health benefits achievable with modest weight loss, delivering comprehensive lifestyle management, ideally at the pre-morbid stage of the condition, is critical.

References

1. Foresight. Tackling Obesities: Future Choices. Project Report. Government Office for Science; 2008.
2. The NHS Information Centre LS. Statistics on Obesity. Activity and Diet: England 2010. The Health and Social Care Information Centre; 2010.
3. Health Survey for England 2009. www.ic.nhs.uk/pubs/hse09report; 2009 [accessed 31.10.11].
4. McPherson K, Marsh T. Modelling Future Trends in Obesity and the Impact on Health. Foresight Tackling Obesities: Future Choices. http://www.bis.gov.uk/foresight; 2007.
5. Health Survey for England 2007. http://www.dh.gov.uk/health/category/publications/; 2007 [accessed 31.10.11].
6. The NHS Information Centre. Statistics on Obesity, Physical Activity and Diet: England 2006.
7. Fontaine KR, Redden DT, Wang C, Westfall AO, Allison DB. Years of life lost due to obesity. JAMA 2003 Jan 8;289[2]:187–93.
8. Manson JE, Willett WC, Stampfer MJ, Colditz GA, Hunter DJ, Hankinson SE. Body weight and mortality among women. N Engl J Med 1995 Sep 14;333[11]:677–85.
9. Calle EE, Rodriguez C, Walker-Thurmond K, Thun MJ. Overweight, obesity, and mortality from cancer in a prospectively studied cohort of US adults. N Engl J Med 2003 Apr 24;348[17]:1625–38.
10. Bender R, Trautner C, Spraul M, Berger M. Assessment of excess mortality in obesity. Am J Epidemiol 1998 Jan 1;147[1]:42–8.
11. Gu D, He J, Duan X, Reynolds K, Wu X, Chen J, et al. Body weight and mortality among men and women in China. JAMA 2006 Feb 15;295[7]:776–83.
12. World Health Organization. Obesity: Preventing and Managing the Global Epidemic. Working Group on Obesity. Geneva: World Health Organization; 1998.
13. Hu FB, Willett WC, Li T, Stampfer MJ, Colditz GA, Manson JE. Adiposity as compared with physical activity in predicting mortality among women. N Engl J Med 2004 Dec 23;351[26]:2694–703.
14. Colditz GA, Willett WC, Stampfer MJ, Manson JE, Hennekens CH, Arky RA, et al. Weight as a risk factor for clinical diabetes in women. Am J Epidemiol 1990 Sep;132[3]:501–13.
15. Colditz GA, Willett WC, Rotnitzky A, Manson JE. Weight gain as a risk factor for clinical diabetes mellitus in women. Ann Intern Med 1995 Apr 1;122[7]:481–6.
16. Wannamethee SG, Shaper AG. Weight change and duration of overweight and obesity in the incidence of type 2 diabetes. Diabetes Care 1999 Aug;22[8]:1266–72.
17. Chan JM, Rimm EB, Colditz GA, Stampfer MJ, Willett WC. Obesity, fat distribution, and weight gain as risk factors for clinical diabetes in men. Diabetes Care 1994 Sep;17[9]:961–9.
18. Martinez ME, Giovannucci E, Spiegelman D, Hunter DJ, Willett WC, Colditz GA. Leisure-time physical activity, body size, and colon cancer in women. Nurses' Health Study Research Group. J Natl Cancer Inst 1997 Jul 2;89[13]:948–55.

19. Giovannucci E, Ascherio A, Rimm EB, Colditz GA, Stampfer MJ, Willett WC. Physical activity, obesity, and risk for colon cancer and adenoma in men. Ann Intern Med 1995 Mar 1;122[5]:327–34.

20. Barakat HA, Carpenter JW, McLendon VD, Khazanie P, Leggett N, Heath J, et al. Influence of obesity, impaired glucose tolerance, and NIDDM on LDL structure and composition. Possible link between hyperinsulinemia and atherosclerosis. Diabetes 1990 Dec;39[12]:1527–33.

21. Hubert HB, Feinleib M, McNamara PM, Castelli WP. Obesity as an independent risk factor for cardiovascular disease: a 26-year follow-up of participants in the Framingham Heart Study. Circulation 1983 May;67[5]:968–77.

22. Manson JE, Colditz GA, Stampfer MJ, Willett WC, Rosner B, Monson RR, et al. A prospective study of obesity and risk of coronary heart disease in women. N Engl J Med 1990 Mar 29;322[13]:882–9.

23. Despres JP. Dyslipidaemia and obesity. Baillieres Clin Endocrinol Metab 1994 Jul;8[3]: 629–60.

24. Kolotkin RL, Meter K, Williams GR. Quality of life and obesity. Obes Rev 2001 Nov;2[4]:219–29.

25. Kushner RF, Foster GD. Obesity and quality of life. Nutrition 2000 Oct; 16[10]:947–52.

26. Luppino FS, de Wit LM, Bouvy PF, Stijnen T, Cuijpers P, Penninx BW, et al. Overweight, obesity, and depression: a systematic review and meta-analysis of longitudinal studies. Arch Gen Psychiatry 2010 Mar;67[3]:220–9.

27. Parsons A, Shraim M, Inglis J, Aveyard P, Hajek P. Interventions for preventing weight gain after smoking cessation. Cochrane Database of Systematic Reviews 2009;Issue 1 (Art. No.: CD006219. DOI: 10.1002/14651858.CD006219.pub2).

28. Pisinger C, Jorgensen T. Waist circumference and weight following smoking cessation in a general population: the Inter99 study. Prev Med 2007 Apr;44[4]:290–5.

29. Scottish Intercollegiate Guidelines Network. Management of Obesity: A National Clinical Guideline; 2010.

30. Gallo M, Lopez L, Grimes D, Schultz K, Helmerhorst F. Combination contraceptives: effects on weight. Cochrane Library; 2006.

31. Rolls ET. Understanding the mechanisms of food intake and obesity. Obes Rev 2007 Mar;8[Suppl. 1]:67–72.

32. Prentice A. Are defects in energy expenditure involved in the causation of obesity? Obes Rev 2007 Mar;8[Suppl. 1]:89–91.

33. Barker DJ. Obesity and early life. Obes Rev 2007 Mar;8[Suppl. 1]:45–9.

34. Avenell A, Broom J, Brown TJ, Poobalan A, Aucott L, Stearns SC, et al. Systematic review of the long-term effects and economic consequences of treatments for obesity and implications for health improvement. Health Technol Assess 2004 May;8[21]:iii–iv, 1–182.

35. Stenius-Aarniala B, Poussa T, Kvarnstrom J, Gronlund EL, Ylikahri M, Mustajoki P. Immediate and long term effects of weight reduction in obese people with asthma: randomised controlled study. BMJ 2000 Mar 25;320[7238]:827–32.

36. Christensen R, Bartels EM, Astrup A, Bliddal H. Effect of weight reduction in obese patients diagnosed with knee osteoarthritis: a systematic review and meta-analysis. Ann Rheum Dis 2007 Apr;66[4]:433–9.

37. Bales CW, Buhr G. Is obesity bad for older persons? A systematic review of the pros and cons of weight reduction in later life. J Am Med Dir Assoc 2008 Jun; 9[5]:302–12.

38. Mulrow CD, Chiquette E, Angel L, Cornell J, Summerbell C, Anagnostelis B. Dieting to reduce body weight for controlling hypertension in adults. Cochrane Library; 2006.
39. Vettor R, Serra R, Fabris R, Pagano C, Federspil G. Effect of sibutramine on weight management and metabolic control in type 2 diabetes: a meta-analysis of clinical studies. Diabetes Care 2005 Apr;28[4]:942–9.
40. McTigue KM, Harris R, Hemphill B, Lux L, Sutton S, Bunton AJ. Screening and interventions for obesity in adults: summary of the evidence for the US Preventive Services Task Force. Ann Intern Med 2003 Dec 2;139[11]:933–49.
41. Poobalan A, Aucott L, Smith WC, Avenell A, Jung R, Broom J. Effects of weight loss in overweight/obese individuals and long-term lipid outcomes – a systematic review. Obes Rev 2004 Feb;5[1]:43–50.

2 Health Professionals' Attitudes Towards Obesity and its Management

Obesity is not a self-inflicted problem which would be cured if only people tried harder and stuck to their diets

---

Consider these comments

'I know no one who isn't guilty of ridiculing a person at least once for being fat. Everyone is guilty of it, and yet nothing is done about it. This "sizism" is the last place where people can discriminate openly without fear of reprimand. We're the last safe prejudice' [1].

'Fat people report they are accosted on the street by strangers who admonish them to lose weight. Often their own children are ashamed of them ... even many doctors find fat people disgusting, and some refuse to treat them' [2].

'When you are obese no one wants to talk to you, no one wants to have you around because you are an embarrassment; of course no "normal" weight person would ever stop to consider how much embarrassment an obese person feels daily' [3].

As health professionals working with obese patients we need to take time to consider these critical issues. What are our attitudes (overt and subtle) to overweight people, how does this impact on our practice, and what can we do to counter weight discrimination and prejudice in health care?

Weight bias is any negative attitude that influences how we interact with overweight and obese people. It can occur in a variety of ways, such as verbal teasing, bullying and aggression, or more subtly through social exclusion, such as being ignored or overlooked. Weight bias often presents as stereotypes, where automatic assumptions are made about a patient based simply on their obesity. Stigma, prejudice and discrimination in health care settings may lead to less time invested in consultations with obese patients, not bothering to raise the issue of weight, making assumptions about why weight loss hasn't occurred, or assuming the cause of a health problem is inevitably weight-related.

Weight Management: A Practitioner's Guide, First Edition. Dympna Pearson and Clare Grace.
© 2012 Dympna Pearson and Clare Grace. Published 2012 by Blackwell Publishing Ltd.

Examples of weight bias

Example 1: Insensitive weighing

'I stopped going to the clinic. I was too heavy for the scales. The nurse raised her eyebrows and told me I'd have to find some industrial scales. I just wanted the ground to open up and swallow me.'

Example 2: Just try harder

'When I went back to see the dietitian she weighed me and said I hadn't lost weight. I tried to tell her how I could not manage the changes we discussed but she didn't listen. She told me I needed to try harder and say "no" to snacks.'

Example 3: All health issues are weight-related

'I've stopped going to my doctor. No matter what my health problem, I'm just told it's because of my weight.'

What does the evidence say about discrimination and weight bias in society?

There is strong scientific evidence supporting the widespread existence of negative attitudes and stereotypes across a range of settings [4].

In employment

- Obese people are less likely to be hired [5] and have lower wages and fewer promotions that non-obese people with comparable qualifications and experience [6].
- Employers and coworkers believe obese colleagues have less self-discipline, less ambition and poor personal hygiene [7].

In education

- Negative attitudes are common in schools and begin in children aged 3–5 years. Research in this age group has shown they associate overweight peers with being stupid, ugly, unhappy, lazy and having few friends [8].
- A third of overweight girls and a quarter of overweight boys report being teased and bullied about their weight in school, which increases to 60% in obese children [9,10]. Weight bias has also been found in teachers [11].
- Obese applicants are less likely to be accepted in college than non-obese applicants with comparable qualifications and academic performance [12].
- *'For fat students, the school experience is one of ongoing prejudice, unnoticed discrimination, and almost constant harassment'* [13].

In health care

- When obese people have been asked to rank who is the most common source of weight bias, doctors are second on their list [4].
- Doctors have reported obese people as weak-willed, noncompliant, lacking in self-control and lazy [14]. Similar beliefs have also been expressed by medical students [15].
- Likewise, nurses report obese patients to be noncompliant, lazy and overindulgent, with over 31% reporting they would prefer not to care for the overweight patient [16,17].
- A survey of UK dietitians suggests neutral to positive attitudes to overweight people, although the obese were viewed less favourably [18]. Earlier research suggests dietitians believe obesity is caused by emotional problems, together with an ambivalence towards management recommendations [19,20].

The evidence above has focused on people's explicit attitudes; that is, they have been directly asked what they think about obese people.

Other research has looked at more subtle indicators to explore weight bias which people may be unaware of, or are unwilling to openly admit, sometimes referred to as implicit attitudes. This research looks either at health professionals' responses to how they would care for hypothetical patients, or at the speed of pairing positive and negative attributes to obese versus lean subjects (implicit association test, Resource 1).

In one study, GPs were sent six hypothetical patients who varied only in their gender and BMI (23, 30, 36 kg/m^2). They were asked to comment on how they would care for each patient (procedures, tests and referrals), how much time they'd spend on consultations, and their emotional and behavioural responses to the patients. Negative attitudes were BMI-dependent, with less investment in obese patients in terms of both consultation time (20–30% less time spent with obese patients) and willingness to help [21].

Research using the implicit association test in professionals specialising in obesity management, who you would assume would be immune from weight bias, have found implicit negative attitudes towards obese people, albeit to a lesser extent than is observed in the lay population [22]. This underlines the importance of not assuming immunity to weight bias due to an expertise in the field.

Where does weight bias come from?

The following factors are thought to be involved in creating and influencing weight bias in society.

Media and TV images

Obese people appear infrequently on TV and in the media and when they do they tend to be in stereotypical roles [23]. This means there are few positive social roles for obese people via the media.

Cultural factors

Being thin in Western society equates to beauty and self-control. It is commonly believed that attaining an ideal shape/size is feasible if only a person is sufficiently self-disciplined.

Beliefs about the causes of obesity

There is a widely held misconception that obesity is entirely within a person's control. So an obese person is led to believe that if they struggle to control their weight, they must be lacking in willpower.

What are the consequences of weight bias?

There are known to be social, psychological and physical consequences of weight bias for obese people.

Psychological consequences

Greater vulnerability for depression, anxiety, low self-esteem and poor body image [10].

Social and economic consequences

Weight bias may impact negatively on social relationships, leading to social rejection and isolation. Bias in educational settings is believed to be one explanation for the lower household incomes of obese individuals observed in some studies [24].

Physical consequences

Weight-related teasing has been linked to extreme weight-control practices and dysfunctional eating in adolescent girls and boys [25]. Some obese adults report responding to stigma by eating more as a way of coping with these negative experiences, others report a defiant response by refusing to change their eating habits in response to weight bias [26].

What is the impact of weight bias in the health care setting?

Although there is strong evidence for the widespread existence of weight bias among health professionals, there is far less research on whether, or how, this impacts on the quality of care and the weight-management consultation. However, the following should be considered:

- Negative attitudes may create an intolerant environment where the obese patient feels blamed rather than supported. This may affect the therapeutic relationship with the practitioner, the patient's experience of the consultation, and probably motivation and self-esteem.
- A health professional who holds negative attitudes may be less prepared to raise the issue of overweight, invest less time in a consultation, provide fewer intervention options and be less prepared to offer certain tests, procedures or referrals.
- Research has shown that obese women take up preventative services less frequently than non-obese and are more likely to delay or cancel an appointment [27,28]. Responsible factors include: disrespect from health professionals, embarrassment about being weighed, medical equipment that is too small, and unsolicited advice to lose weight [29]. The experience, or anticipation, of weight bias during a consultation may partially explain the high rates of nonattendance seen in weight-management programmes.
- A vicious cycle in obesity has been described where obese people use health services frequently due to obesity co-morbidities, but the weight bias experienced leads to avoidance of health care, poor management of their condition and further exacerbation of their disease [30].
- Poor commissioning of services may occur if those involved in awarding funding hold negative views on obesity, its causes and management.

What can we do to reduce weight bias?

- Evidence supports the widespread existence of negative attitudes towards obesity in health professionals, even those specialising in weight management. Therefore it is important we honestly evaluate our attitudes to obesity and take steps to address any stereotyping negatively affecting our practice.
- Presented below are some common scenarios. Consider how you might respond and whether you might make some unhelpful assumptions. It is also possible to explore your levels of subtle weight bias by taking the implicit association test (Resource 1). It takes approximately 15 minutes to complete.
- Check out the 'exposing weight bias' educational videos available at the Rudd Center (Resource 2).

Conclusion

As health practitioners, we are probably all guilty, to a greater or lesser extent, of weight bias. It is important to reflect on our attitudes, be aware of the widespread nature of weight bias in society and consider how our practice can be adjusted to improve the quality of care and the patient's experience of treatment.

Reflective exercises

Consider the scenarios below and reflect on how you might feel and behave in these situations.

Scenario 1

You're standing in the supermarket queue and in front of you is an obese woman. Do you look in her trolley to check what she's buying? If her trolley contains high-calorie snack foods and sugary drinks, do you have thoughts about how that might be influencing her weight? Would your thoughts and reactions be different if the trolley full of high-calorie foods were being pushed by a slim woman?

Scenario 2

You're sitting on the bus on a very hot day and it is crowded. All the seats are filling up and now the only seat left is next to you. A hot and bothered obese man is clearly looking for a seat. What might your thoughts be? Would you feel differently if the man were slim?

Scenario 3

You're driving down the road and you see a very large woman in keep-fit gear jogging slowly. She looks very out of breath and is clearly finding it hard work. What might your thoughts be? Would you think differently if the woman were slim and fit?

Consider these clinical scenarios:

Scenario 1

A 35-year-old obese woman with a BMI of 42 kg/m^2 is returning for a follow-up appointment. You spent a long time at the first appointment discussing treatment options and she seemed motivated to change her habits. You agreed a 2 lb weight-loss goal but she's gained 1 lb.

What is your immediate reaction to this news? What are your thoughts about why this has happened? Do you question whether she has tried hard enough or has inadequate willpower? How do you proceed with the consultation? Do you decide to invest less time in this patient? How would you rate her chances of succeeding with her weight-loss attempts?

Scenario 2

In the following, consider:

- What assumptions is the doctor making?
- What effect might this have on the patient's motivation to change?
- How might things have been done differently?

Mrs X has made an appointment to see her doctor as she's keen to lose weight. Her father died recently from the complications of diabetes and this has dramatically increased her motivation to reduce her own risk. She thinks her doctor will be able to advise her on the best way to achieve this.

Doctor: *'What can I do for you today, Mrs X?'*
Mrs X: *'Well, I've decided I really need to lose weight and I wanted your advice.'*
Doctor: *'Well, Mrs X, I'm delighted to hear you have finally decided to sort out your weight. It really is too high – you are in the red section of the BMI chart, meaning you are obese, and this puts you at much higher risk of heart disease, diabetes and cancer. Now, to lose weight you need to eat less calories and burn off more through exercise. So cut out all those biscuits, cakes and crisps and swap to diet fizzy drinks. Exercise is essential too, so maybe join a gym.'*

The doctor assumes:

1 Mrs X doesn't know the risks associated with her weight. If her reasons for wanting to lose weight had been explored, her awareness of the connection between overweight and risk of diabetes would have been identified.
2 The source of excess calories is from biscuits, cakes, crisps and fizzy drinks and she is currently inactive, even though none of these issues are explored.

In this scenario the patient is unlikely to feel listened to and this may have a negative impact on her motivation.

Recommendations for reducing weight bias in your practice

- Be aware that many obese patients will have made numerous previous attempts to lose weight. If this is the case, it is important to acknowledge the time and effort that they have already invested in trying to address their obesity.
- Acknowledge the various and complex causes of obesity. If appropriate, highlight that science shows some people are more predisposed to struggle with their weight than others. Acknowledge that managing weight is not a simple process and presents an ongoing, but not insurmountable, challenge.
- Be aware of the sensitivity around weighing. Ask patients for permission to check their weight and, if they agree, ensure this is done in private with no negative comments or facial gestures made in response to the reading. Ensure there are scales that will weigh people up to 250 kg (300+ kg in bariatric patients).
- Ensure the consultation and waiting rooms have appropriate facilities, e.g. seating without arms, large blood-pressure cuffs, large gowns.

References

1. Lampert L. Fat like me. Ladies Home Journal 1993 May:154–215.
2. Flanagan SA. Obesity: the last bastion of prejudice. Obes Surg 1996 Oct;6[5]:430–7.
3. Kolata G. Are fat people last to beat bias? Eugene Register Guard 1992.

4. Puhl R, Brownell KD. Bias, discrimination, and obesity. Obes Res 2001 Dec;9[12]: 788–805.
5. Pingitore R, Dugoni R, Tindale S, Spring B. Bias against overweight job applicants in a simulated employment interview. J Appl Psychol 1997;79:909–17.
6. Pagan J, Davila A. Obesity, occupational attainment and earnings. Social Science Quarterly 1997;78:756–70.
7. Roehling M. Weight-biased discrimination in employment: psychological and legal aspects. Personnel Psychol 1999;52:969–1017.
8. Cramer P, Steinwert T. Thin is good, fat is bad: how early does it begin? Journal of Applied Developmental Psychology 1998;19:429–51.
9. Griffiths LJ, Wolke D, Page AS, Horwood JP. Obesity and bullying: different effects for boys and girls. Arch Dis Child 2006 Feb;91[2]:121–5.
10. Eisenberg ME, Neumark-Sztainer D, Story M. Associations of weight-based teasing and emotional well-being among adolescents. Arch Pediatr Adolesc Med 2003 Aug;157[8]:733–8.
11. Neumark-Sztainer D, Story M, Harris T. Beliefs and attitudes about obesity among teachers & school healthcare providers working with adolescents. Journal of Nutrition Education 1999;31[1]:3–9.
12. Karnehed N, Rasmussen F, Hemmingsson T, Tynelius P. Obesity and attained education: cohort study of more than 700,000 Swedish men. Obesity (Silver Spring) 2006 Aug;14[8]:1421–8.
13. National Education Association. Report on Discrimination due to Physical Size. Washington, DC: National Education Association; 1994.
14. Campbell K, Engel H, Timperio A, Cooper C, Crawford D. Obesity management: Australian general practitioners' attitudes and practices. Obes Res 2000 Sep;8[6]: 459–66.
15. Wigton RS, McGaghie WC. The effect of obesity on medical students' approach to patients with abdominal pain. J Gen Intern Med 2001 Apr;16[4]:262–5.
16. Hoppe R, Ogden J. Practice nurses' beliefs about obesity and weight related interventions in primary care. Int J Obes Relat Metab Disord 1997 Feb;21[2]:141–6.
17. Maroney D, Golub S. Nurses' attitudes toward obese persons and certain ethnic groups. Percept Mot Skills 1992 Oct;75[2]:387–91.
18. Harvey EL, Summerbell CD, Kirk SF, Hill AJ. Dietitians' views of overweight and obese people and reported management practices. J Hum Nutr Diet 2002 Oct;15[5]:331–47.
19. McArthur LH, Ross JK. Attitudes of registered dietitians toward personal overweight and overweight patients. J Am Diet Assoc 1997 Jan;97[1]:63–6.
20. Oberrieder H, Walker R, Monroe D, Adeyanju M. Attitude of dietetics students and registered dietitians toward obesity. J Am Diet Assoc 1995 Aug;95[8]:914–6.
21. Hebl MR, Xu J. Weighing the care: physicians' reactions to the size of a patient. Int J Obes Relat Metab Disord 2001 Aug;25[8]:1246–52.
22. Teachman BA, Brownell KD. Implicit anti-fat bias among health professionals: is anyone immune? Int J Obes Relat Metab Disord 2001 Oct;25[10]:1525–31.
23. Greenberg BS, Eastin M, Hofshire L, Lachlan K, Brownell KD. Portrayals of overweight and obese individuals on commercial television. Am J Public Health 2003 Aug;93[8]:1342–8.
24. Gortmaker SL, Must A, Perrin JM, Sobol AM, Dietz WH. Social and economic consequences of overweight in adolescence and young adulthood. N Engl J Med 1993 Sep 30;329[14]:1008–12.

25. Haines J, Neumark-Sztainer D, Eisenberg ME, Hannan PJ. Weight teasing and disordered eating behaviors in adolescents: longitudinal findings from Project EAT (Eating Among Teens). Pediatrics 2006 Feb;117[2]:e209–15.

26. Puhl RM, Brownell KD. Confronting and coping with weight stigma: an investigation of overweight and obese adults. Obesity (Silver Spring) 2006 Oct;14[10]:1802–15.

27. Adams CH, Smith NJ, Wilbur DC, Grady KE. The relationship of obesity to the frequency of pelvic examinations: do physician and patient attitudes make a difference? Women Health 1993;20[2]:45–57.

28. Drury CA, Louis M. Exploring the association between body weight, stigma of obesity, and health care avoidance. J Am Acad Nurse Pract 2002 Dec;14[12]:554–61.

29. Amy NK, Aalborg A, Lyons P, Keranen L. Barriers to routine gynecological cancer screening for White and African-American obese women. Int J Obes (Lond) 2006 Jan; 30[1]:147–55.

30. Brownell KD, Puhl R, Schwartz M, Rudd L, editors. Weight Bias: Nature, Consequences and Remedies. Guilford Pubn; 2005.

3 Treatment Options: The Evidence for What Works

'It ain't what people don't know that hurts them it's what they know that ain't so.'

Mark Twain

Introduction

Given the desperation to lose weight experienced by some patients it is unsurprising that large amounts of money, time and effort are invested in strategies which may not be supported by evidence for their efficacy and safety. Such approaches can detract people from focusing on the key changes required for long-term weight management. Repeated failed attempts to manage weight may have a detrimental effect on a person's belief that weight loss is feasible. Part of the health professional's role is to guide patients towards scientifically safe and effective treatments.

This chapter summarises current evidence (at the time of publication) for common treatment approaches and highlights areas where further research is required. For some treatments it guides the reader to additional sources of information.

Combined approaches

Weight-loss outcomes are improved when diet, physical activity and behaviour modification are combined, hence the recommendation for multicomponent interventions [1,2]. Although this is well recognised, in reality it is often poorly practised. This may, in part, be due to a lack of understanding on how best to combine, and deliver, evidence-based interventions which meet the needs of the patient. Part 2 of this book considers practical approaches to addressing these challenges. This chapter outlines treatment approaches underpinned by sound evidence and highlights those which require further research prior to recommendation.

Weight Management: A Practitioner's Guide, First Edition. Dympna Pearson and Clare Grace.
© 2012 Dympna Pearson and Clare Grace. Published 2012 by Blackwell Publishing Ltd.

Dietary treatments

Eating frequency and patterns

Erratic eating is a common practice in overweight and obese patients and may range from skipped meals and long periods without eating to grazing, frequent snacking and binge eating. It may relate to years of inappropriate dieting, or may be a misguided means of managing weight. Much of the evidence on eating frequency and weight control is drawn from cross-sectional studies and more research is required before definitive recommendations on an optimal meal pattern can be made. However, skipping breakfast has been associated with an increased risk of obesity in a number of studies [3–5] and those individuals successfully preventing weight regain are more likely to be regular breakfast eaters [6]. Regular breakfast consumption may be beneficial through its influence on reducing impulsive snacking and reduced food intake at subsequent meals [7,8]. In its position paper on weight management, the American Dietetic Association suggests four or five meals/snacks per day (including breakfast) [9], spread throughout the day. This is based on the evidence that four or five meals/snacks per day is associated with the lowest obesity risk compared to irregular eating (three or less meals/snacks per day) or high-frequency eating (more than six meals/snacks per day) [10,11].

Improving the quality of the diet

Helping patients move towards a healthier diet is important for several reasons. Improving the intake of fruits, vegetables and whole grains and modifying fatty acid composition is known to have a beneficial impact on risk factors for cardiovascular health, type 2 diabetes and certain types of cancer, independent of weight loss [12–14]. Second, there is growing evidence to suggest the obese population is at greater risk of vitamin and mineral deficiencies compared to the general population; in one study, 48.7% of patients awaiting bariatric surgery were found to have at least one of the most common micronutrient deficiencies [15]. Vitamin D deficiency is the most prevalent, with research suggesting 25–80% of very obese patients awaiting bariatric surgery are deficient [15,16]. Although it seems paradoxical that an overconsumption of calories could occur in parallel with an inadequate intake of micronutrients, serious vitamin and mineral deficiencies are found in the obese, and poor diet quality may be one possible explanation.

Low-fat diets

Low-fat diets are the prime dietary treatment. Reducing dietary fat usually (but not always) lowers calorie intake, as well as having a beneficial impact on risk reduction for cardiovascular disease. To date, three meta-analyses have examined the effect of ad libitum (no calorie restriction advised) low-fat diets on weight change in lean, overweight and obese subjects. Fat restriction alone seems to be an effective method of lowering energy density (calorie concentration) and is associated with spontaneous weight loss. A 10% reduction of dietary fat leads to ~3–4 kg weight loss in normal–overweight subjects and ~5–6 kg weight loss in the obese [17]. However, it remains unclear whether advising a low-fat diet plus an overall calorie restriction provides improved weight-loss outcomes compared to low-fat diets without advice on calorie restriction. Nonetheless, it seems prudent to convey to patients that although restricting fat intake can automatically produce weight loss, it is not uncommon for conscious, or unconscious, changes in other aspects of food intake to occur.

The 600 kcal deficit approach

Traditionally, diets with fixed calorie levels have been advised: 1500 kcal for women and 1800 kcal for men. Although these are helpful for some, the larger the patient, the greater the challenge, as the difference between their calorie needs and their calorie prescription will be higher. It has been suggested that modest reductions in calories consumed (500–600 kcal) from baseline levels may be more sustainable [18]. Reducing calorie intake by 500–600 kcal each day equates to a 3500 kcal deficit over 7 days, equivalent to a 0.5 kg/1 lb weight loss. This is an approach commonly used by dieticians and involves predicting the patient's base metabolic rate, multiplying this by a factor that takes account of their physical-activity level and then subtracting 600 kcal. This provides an individualised calorie prescription for weight loss and can be translated into practical food choices and number of servings from various food groups.

The 600 kcal deficit approach has been demonstrated to be an effective strategy for some individuals, with a review of 13 randomised controlled trials showing a weight loss of 5.32 kg compared with usual care at 12 months [19]. These diets are in line with the dietary recommendations for good health [20], focusing on a low-fat, higher-complex-carbohydrate intake.

Meal replacements

Meal replacements are portion-controlled products that are vitamin- and mineral-fortified and replace one or two meals in the day, allowing one low-calorie meal using standard foods (and snack(s)) [21]. They often come in the form of milkshakes, meal bars or soups, with two meal replacements and one healthy meal each day providing about 1200–1600 kcal per day. This approach should not be confused with very-low-calorie diets, where all meals and snacks are replaced with the diet product and calorie intake is below 800 kcal/day.

Traditionally, health professionals have given little attention to meal replacements in the management of obesity. However, a number of recent studies have suggested this may be a promising intervention. The special interest group of the British

Dietetic Association (DOM UK) has produced a position paper which summarises the short- and longer-term evidence for the effectiveness of meal replacements (www.domuk.org). In brief, it concludes there is sufficient evidence to support their use as one of a range of possible dietary treatments for the management of overweight and obesity. A number of studies have demonstrated the short-term effectiveness of meal replacements, showing them to be at least as effective as conventional dietary treatment, with some suggestion they may encourage weight maintenance when one meal-replacement product is used each day. Most studies have used meal replacements as part of a comprehensive management programme, with support and education from health professionals, though little is known about the value of their 'off-the-shelf' use without health-professional support. More information is needed on the type of patient that responds well to this dietary treatment, and how to integrate meal replacements in UK health care and community settings. Little is known about how effective this type of dietary treatment will prove in obese people with a BMI >45 kg/m^2 as studies to date have included subjects in lower BMI categories. These recommendations are in line with those from the American Dietetic Association, which concluded 'for people who have difficulty with self-selection and/or portion control, meal replacements may be used as part of the diet component of a comprehensive weight management program. Substituting one or two daily meals or snacks with meal replacements is a successful weight loss and weight maintenance strategy' [22].

Very-low-calorie diets

Very-low-calorie diets (VLCDs) are a total replacement for all meals and snacks and provide 450–800 kcal/day [23,24]. There is no doubt that such an extreme energy restriction leads to substantial short-term weight loss, but weight regain is common. It is unclear from the available research whether long-term outcomes with VLCDs are better than those achieved with more conventional dietary treatments. However, for approximately 25–35% of people treated with a VLCD, modest weight loss will still be evident 2–7 years later [25], suggesting that for a small, and carefully selected group, this may be a helpful strategy.

Given the extent of calorie restriction and their associated risks, VLCDs should not be used as a first-line dietary treatment and are best reserved for use in patients with BMI ≥30 kg/m^2 with medical conditions likely to benefit from rapid weight loss. It is recommended that continuous use of VLCDs should be limited to 12 weeks and requires close medical supervision [2]. To improve weight maintenance, VLCDs should be used as part of a comprehensive management package in which strategies to support maintenance (e.g. cognitive behavioural therapy (CBT), pharmacotherapy) after the food-reintroduction phase have been considered. DOM UK has produced a position paper which summarises short-term and longer-term evidence for VLCD use in obesity management, highlights areas of uncertainty in the literature, and discusses how these relate to their use in practice (Resource 3).

Example of VLCD monitoring requirements

Medical monitoring
- medical history and examination
- assessment of disordered eating behaviour
- thyroid function test, full blood count, electrolytes, lipid profile, glucose, insulin, renal and liver function
- recent ECG if uncertainty about cardiac function
- side effects monitored and medication adjusted.

Every 1–2 weeks
- weight, BP and pulse check.

Dietetic support
- fortnightly
- high-input during food-reintroduction phase
- link with pharmacotherapy and/or CBT.

Low-glycaemic-index diets

The glycaemic index (GI) is a way of ranking carbohydrate foods depending on the speed of their absorption. Low-GI foods are absorbed more slowly than high-GI foods and this may influence appetite control through reduced hyperglycaemia and hyperinsulinaemia after meals. Glycaemic load (GL) is a newer concept which accounts for the GI of a food as well as the carbohydrate in the *portion size* of the food in question, with some suggesting this is a better reflection of the glycaemic response to mixed meals [26–28].

Whether low-GI or GL diets are an effective weight-management treatment remains a hotly debated issue among nutritionists [29–31]. Advocates of the low-GI approach argue that high-carbohydrate, low-fat diets may increase hyperglycaemia and hyperinsulinaemia after meals, making weight loss more challenging, as carbohydrate is used at the expense of fat, leading to increased fat storage [29]. Although there is some interesting evidence from animal research, studies in humans have been mixed [32]. Shortfalls in the quality of the human research raise doubts over the conclusion that a low-GI diet is superior to a low-fat, high-carbohydrate diet for weight management in healthy overweight people [32].

A recent Cochrane review explored low-GI and low-GL diets and their role in weight management and found an improved weight loss (~1 kg greater) in those on low-GI compared to control diets [33]. However, the dietary interventions were short-term (5 weeks to 6 months), with a limited follow-up period, and with most of the studies not including overweight and obese participants. There is a need for long-term studies with sufficient numbers of participants, and using well-controlled diets, in order to truly understand the impact of this approach in weight management. As such, it seems premature to routinely recommend this strategy as an evidence-based weight-loss approach [9] until the results for large-scale, long-term randomised controlled trials have become available. However, low-GI and GL diets do promote higher intakes of whole grains, which are known to have beneficial health effects and may be of value in risk reduction. Recent research on weight maintenance suggests lower GI diets may be helpful in preventing weight re-gain [34].

Low-carbohydrate diets

Low-carbohydrate, high-protein diets have proved a popular weight-loss approach, although their efficacy and safety remain controversial. Diets such as Atkins and Protein Power typically contain a high proportion of protein foods (~35% energy), unrestricted use of fats (>50% energy), particularly saturated fats, and a severe restriction on carbohydrates (<10% energy). Evidence from randomised controlled trials suggests improved weight loss over the short term with low-carbohydrate diets, but studies are small and drop-out is high [35]. The long-term (>1 year) health effects of low-carbohydrate diets are unknown in terms of cardiovascular health, renal function, bone health and cancer risk [36], especially in those with obesity-related diseases. Evidence of nutritional shortfalls has also been recorded [37].

Currently there is no scientific consensus on the optimal macronutrient composition for weight management. There is growing interest in the potential for substituting a proportion of dietary energy from carbohydrate with protein while retaining a low-fat intake. Such diets are different from the popular high-protein diets, being lower in protein (~25%E), much lower in fat (<30%E) and higher in carbohydrate (~40%). Early research suggests this approach may be beneficial in the short term, although beyond 1 year major benefits seem to be lost [38] and there is a need for more research before amendments to advice occur. However, for weight maintenance, modest increase to protein seems to improve weight maintenance outcomes, although the effect beyond 6 months is unclear [34].

Fad diets

Unfortunately, there are a huge number of 'fad' weight loss diets (e.g. detox, food combining, blood group diet, etc.) that are not supported by scientific evidence in terms of their efficacy and/or safety. They make enticing promises about the speed and ease of weight loss and may advocate dietary and lifestyle approaches out of line with current scientific thinking [39]. They detract from appropriate methods of managing weight and confuse people on what are helpful approaches (see Chapter 7 for more).

Physical-activity treatments

In weight management, promotion of physical activity should have equal billing with dietary change. However, in reality, activity promotion is often the forgotten component [40].

Using physical activity as a sole intervention to manage obesity is associated with disappointing outcomes [1,41,42] and diet is recognised as a more potent weight-loss treatment [43]. It is very challenging to quickly induce the 500–1000 calorie deficit needed each day for a 0.5–1 kg loss per week. This 'dose' of activity is usually beyond the physical ability of most overweight and obese patients. However, combining activity with dietary change improves weight loss outcomes [2] and has clear benefits for co-morbidity management [44]. For example, improvements to blood lipids and blood pressure occur with regular activity, even if no improvements to weight occur [44,45].

There is also a strong association between the level of physical activity and the prevention of weight regain, although the amount of activity required seems to be high. Emphasising the importance that physical activity plays in weight maintenance can be illustrated by highlighting the findings from the US National Weight Control Registry. This is a database for people who have lost large amounts of weight (mean weight loss 13.5 kg/30 lb) and successfully maintained a substantially reduced weight for at least 1 year. The majority of database members report regular exercise as a key element of their maintenance programme, expending ~2700 calories per week (60–90 minutes activity/day) [45].

More specifically, regular physical activity has been shown to:

- Reduce mortality [46].
- Prevent weight gain and regain [47–49].
- Promote numerous health benefits (e.g. improved blood lipids and blood pressure) even if no weight loss occurs [50,51].
- Possibly reverse early insulin resistance, thereby reducing the risks of developing type 2 diabetes [52] or improving the management of blood glucose in those with diabetes [53].
- Improve weight-loss outcomes when combined with dietary treatments [1].
- Impact positively on self-esteem, physical self-worth, body image and mood [54]. This may influence the individual's capacity to cope with dietary change [55], and the beneficial impact seems to be greater in those with low baseline self-esteem [56].
- Reduce stress levels, anxiety and depression, leading to improved general well being and improved sleep patterns [57].
- Have possible beneficial effects on body composition by limiting the loss of muscle tissue that occurs during weight loss [58].
- Improve functional capacity, mobility and quality of life through increased fitness and muscle strength [59].

How much activity is needed?

The amount of activity recommended depends on weight-management goals [60]. If the goal is:

- Risk reduction for chronic disease:
  - adults should aim to be active daily. Activity should add up to at least 150 minutes per week of moderate-intensity activity in bouts of 10 minutes or more – one way to approach this is to do 30 minutes on at least 5 days per week [61,62].

- Active weight management or prevention of weight gain:
  - 60 minutes of moderate- to vigorous-intensity activity is needed on most days of the week [63].
- Prevention of weight regain after weight loss:
  - 60–90 minutes of daily moderate-intensity physical activity is recommended [63].

Research suggests that the likelihood of achieving these higher doses of physical activity can be improved by incorporating additional support such as the inclusion of family members or the use of group-support sessions with coaches [64].

Intensity and type of activity

There is some debate over the optimal intensity of exercise for managing weight. It has been suggested that activities of vigorous intensity are associated with improved weight-loss outcomes compared to moderate to light activities. However, a recent review found this additional benefit of vigorous activity was only observed when the intensity of exercise was tested without any dietary treatment. When dietary change was added, the intensity of the exercise did not appear to make a difference to weight-loss outcomes, although high-intensity activity may be linked to a greater accrual of associated health benefits [1].

NICE recommends a variety of different physical-activity interventions depending on the preferences of the patient as well as their physical fitness and ability [2].

Interventions should include:

Reduction in sedentary behaviour

This includes limiting time spent watching television or sat in front of the computer. Although this is a popular strategy in managing children's weight, evidence supporting its efficacy in adults is limited. Nevertheless, it is recognised to be a useful starting point for patients with substantial functional limitations, who may struggle to undertake any light-intensity activity.

Increase in activities of daily living

There are a number of studies comparing the effectiveness of lifestyle activity (e.g. walking rather than using transport) to structured exercise. Project Active compared lifestyle activity to structured gym-based exercise programmes with a 6-month intensive-treatment period, followed by 18 months of maintenance with minimal contact. Both groups had comparable improvements in their fitness and body composition and it was concluded that the two strategies were equally effective in improving activity levels and fitness. The weight-loss outcomes were poor in both groups, which was to be expected, as the main focus of the intervention was activity rather than dietary treatments [65]. However, at 1 year significantly less weight had been regained in the lifestyle group compared to the structured group, suggesting lifestyle activity may be important in weight maintenance [66]. Walking is a commonly recommended activity in obese patients, often suiting their physical capabilities. It involves no financial outlay and is usually not associated with negative experiences linked to sports.

Structured exercise

This is the activity people assume must be undertaken, and for some obese patients it may suit their preferences and physical abilities. Structured exercise can often be undertaken in groups, which, for those responsive to group support, can be a useful strategy to consider.

Exercise-on-referral schemes

Referral of sedentary patients by their GP to supervised exercise sessions, run through local leisure facilities, would seem an excellent approach to promoting increased physical activity. However, a systematic review of research suggests that although a little increase in activity is observed in these schemes, the effect is small. A total of 17 patients would need to be treated in order for 1 patient to become moderately active and it has been questioned whether this is a cost-effective use of resources [67]. The limited efficacy of exercise-on-referral schemes seems to relate to poor participation and high attrition. There have been some suggestions this relates to barriers such as poor body image, time-management issues, lack of social support and intimidating activity environments, although more qualitative research is required to develop a better understanding of the reasons for poor participation [67].

Behaviour modification

Evidence consistently shows that combining dietary changes, physical activity and behavioural modification leads to greater weight loss than diet alone. A meta-analysis of five studies found median weight change was −4.8 kg in the combined approaches versus −0.48 kg in the diet alone groups [2]. The use of behavioural approaches in managing weight in those with, or at risk of, type 2 diabetes is also beneficial [68]. In two small studies, low-calorie diet plus behaviour therapy resulted in a 7.7 kg loss versus 0.9 kg loss in low-calorie diet alone [2].

An integrated approach

Although behaviour modification is often discussed as a separate set of strategies tagged on to diet and activity treatments, the behavioural approach to managing weight should extend far beyond a set of techniques. It should influence the whole philosophy of the consultation, together with the skills and perspective of the health professional.

The approach should focus on patient-centred care that incorporates motivational, behavioural and cognitive elements, while acknowledging that the attitudes and skills of the practitioner will have a profound effect on the outcomes of treatment. This is a rather different approach to the traditional advice-giving and persuasion role that is central to traditional treatment, which may increase patient resistance by reducing the individual's involvement and control over the process of change [69].

Traditional weight management tends to follow the medical model of care, with the practitioner as the expert conveying information and the patient as the passive recipient. As behavioural approaches to managing weight have emerged, this approach has been challenged, with the importance of empowerment and patient-centred care being highlighted. Empowerment views the patient as responsible for their own health care and choices, and necessitates practitioners altering their own attitudes to management. The patient and practitioner should be seen as equal and active partners in the consultation process, with the patient as the expert on their own life and the practitioner as the expert on the chronic disease [70]. Indeed, it has been suggested that in order for practitioners to work in this way they need to change their own view of their role by moving away from feeling responsible *for* patients towards being responsible *to* them [71]. Essentially the empowerment approach centres on patient choice, patient responsibility and skills development, and by definition it is also patient-centred. Patient-centred care focuses on involving patients in the decision-making process and tailoring treatment interventions to meet their needs and personal preferences [72]. This approach has been described as the practitioner 'actively seeking to enter into the patient's world to understand his or her unique experiences' [73]. The key principles include the modification of current behaviour patterns, new adaptive learning, problem-solving and a collaborative relationship between patient and therapist [74].

The interpersonal skills of the practitioner are critically important both to the patient's experience of the consultation and the outcomes of treatment. Indeed, a number of behavioural experts have suggested that the practitioner's interpersonal skills are the most potent influencer of change [69,75]. It has been suggested that health professionals will find it very challenging to truly adopt a patient-centred approach without specific and comprehensive training [76].

Key strategies

Outlined below is the evidence supporting some of the individual behavioural components in changing weight-related behaviour.

Self-monitoring

Food diaries are one form of self-monitoring and as suggested earlier, they are a key tool in the assessment of current eating behaviour. Indeed, it has been suggested that if only one skill is conveyed to patients during the whole treatment process, it should be self-monitoring [77]. Individuals who consistently self-monitor have been shown to be more successful in behavioural weight-management programmes compared to those that fail to undertake this strategy [77,78]. The use of diaries is one of the behaviours employed by the successful weight-loss maintainers in the National Weight Control Registry [79]. A willingness to self-monitor and observe their own behaviour often indicates a willingness to come to terms with the eating and activity habits associated with weight control and to subsequently make changes [80].

As patients begin to observe their own behaviours and raise their awareness of how eating and activity behaviours are linked with their weight control, this can, at times, be sufficient to elicit change. This can be further enhanced through working with the practitioner to identify patterns (e.g. long periods without eating, eating in response to stress) that may need to be addressed in treatment. Self-awareness and identification of patterns and behaviours are the key purpose of food and activity diaries and the known level of inaccuracy in the quantification of nutrient intake is of limited relevance. As self-monitoring raises awareness, this can be the first step in the problem-solving process, used to identify the 'problem' in question.

Although self-monitoring is a time-intensive skill, some patients may choose to use it constantly throughout treatment and maintenance. However, for others this might produce 'diary fatigue' and they may choose to use this strategy intermittently, particularly at times when lapses have occurred.

Checking changes in body weight is also a form of self-monitoring, with frequent weight checks seeming to be important to treatment and maintenance success [81]. Daily weighing has been suggested as an important strategy in long-term weight maintenance [82]. This probably relates to the importance of early identification of lapses and subsequent changes to eating and activity behaviour.

Stimulus control

This is a technique that involves the practitioner working with the patient to identify and then develop ways of modifying the cues or the barriers that are linked with unhealthy eating and activity habits. Exposure to cues that are usually associated with a particularly unhelpful behaviour can be linked with relapse, so modifying those cues (stimulus control) can be a helpful approach for many patients [81]. For example, an unhelpful behaviour might be eating dinner in front of the TV. Eating while preoccupied with another activity often reduces the level of awareness of foods consumed or limits the associated satisfaction from the meal. Sitting in front of the TV at other times of the day may subsequently trigger cravings to eat as the patient normally associates TV watching with eating. Breaking this pattern and removing the stimulus by changing the location of meals to the kitchen table with no TV watching may prove useful to improving overall eating behaviour.

Problem-solving

Problem-solving is at the heart of behavioural weight management and is a critical skill for patients to acquire. Part of the health professional's role is to coach and encourage the development of this skill. It can help patients learn how best to cope with various social and emotional situations which will inevitably challenge their newly adopted behaviours. Indeed, it can be these very situations that trigger a lapse, and ultimately a relapse, unless they become skilled and confident in finding alternative ways of handling them. In some instances, patients may attempt to avoid social events that involve eating, but clearly in the long term this is not a feasible management solution and risks socially isolating the patient. Essentially, problem-solving is about helping patients to initially identify the problematic social or emotional situations and then consider a range of possible solutions. From this range of solutions, the patient chooses the one they feel most able to implement, and subsequently evaluate the outcome of this choice. Refinements of the solutions can then be developed or one of the original alternative solutions considered if the outcome was not desirable (see Chapter 7 for more).

Social support

It has been shown that those people with higher levels of social support tend to do better in weight management compared to those with little support [83]. Social support comes in various guises from family members, friends, peers, group programmes or other social activities. It is thought to be important due to its influence on people's sense of motivation and self-efficacy and it may help people become more self-accepting [81]. The right type of social support can also be an invaluable source of positive reinforcement for behavioural goals achieved. However, it should not be assumed that involvement of family members or friends in weight management programmes will automatically have a positive influence, as it will depend on the type of support provided and whether the patient finds this helpful or unhelpful. The attitudes and practices of family, friends and work colleagues can have a positive or negative influence on a patient's weight management efforts, and the strength of the external influence of others varies from one patient to another. Positive support may be in the form of appropriate praise for habits changed or the adoption of supportive behaviours, such as the whole family changing their eating in line with those of the overweight patient. Alternatively, partners, family members or friends may have hindered previous weight-loss attempts through criticism of foods consumed, deliberately offering high-calorie foods or undermining achievements. Identifying the sources and types of helpful and unhelpful support will be the important first stage in developing strategies for establishing a strong network of helpful support (see Chapter 8). It may be important to include a relative as part of a treatment session if they appear to be a substantial barrier to managing weight [84].

Self-rewards

If patients can develop the skill of rewarding themselves for achieving behavioural goals, they are more likely to succeed in maintaining their weight losses at 12 months compared to those that do not self-reward [85,86]. Although this sounds like a relatively straightforward task, for many overweight and obese patients it can be a struggle to identify experiences or objects that they feel comfortable about and which are not food-related. Discussing with patients the types of rewards they have used in previous weight-loss attempts and how they have used rewards can be an enlightening process for both patient and practitioner. It is not unusual for patients never to have thought about how they intend to acknowledge goals achieved and/ or to have a very limited range of rewards, which may be heavily food-focused. It is important to ensure rewards are related to achieving behavioural goals in order to help establish new habits, rather than focusing on weight outcomes. Understanding more about the patient's attitudes and practices in relation to rewards will give an indication of how some of these areas may need to be addressed in treatment.

Drug treatment

Drug treatment has an important role in the management of obesity and may be appropriate after a period of comprehensive lifestyle treatment if the 5–10% weight loss target has not been achieved. However, pharmacotherapy must be prescribed alongside, rather than instead of, lifestyle treatment. Research has shown that providing high-quality diet and activity treatment together with pharmacotherapy leads to improved weight loss compared to medication alone [87]. Despite this evidence, in practice it is common for medication to be used without appropriate dietary treatment. Indeed, one study found only 40% of patients treated with orlistat in primary care had been guided on how to reduce fat intake [88].

Unfortunately, the range of available medications for weight management has declined over recent years, and orlistat is the only prescribable medication in the UK. Orlistat is a pancreatic and gastric lipase inhibitor which prevents 30% of ingested dietary fat from being hydrolysed; this undigested fat is subsequently excreted in the faeces. If orlistat is taken without restriction of dietary fat (30% or less of total calorie intake), side effects of loose oily stool, flatulence and spotting will occur as too much fat is excreted in the faeces.

Orlistat supports weight management in a number of different ways:

1   It facilitates change in the amount of dietary fat in the diet to prevent side effects, thereby lowering total calorie intake.
2   Additional calories are lost via the unabsorbed fat excreted from the body.
3   Eating foods too high in fat leads to unpleasant side effects, which act as a disincentive to eat such foods in the future, theoretically improving motivation to continue eating a low-fat diet.

Orlistat is indicated in patients with a BMI $\geq 30\,kg/m^2$ or $\geq 28\,kg/m^2$ with associated conditions likely to respond to weight loss [2]. It works best in those with a diet high in fat at baseline and which is amenable to fat restriction, but will have little effect in those already following a very-low-fat diet. Hence comprehensive dietary assessment prior to starting drug treatment is important in deciding whether drug treatment is appropriate. As orlistat is minimally absorbed systemically and does not act in the central nervous system, there are few contraindications. However, it shouldn't be used in patients with chronic malabsorption syndrome or cholestasis, or in those who are pregnant or breastfeeding [2].

Orlistat plus lifestyle modification would be expected to produce a weight loss of 5% within 12 weeks. If this is not achieved, NICE recommends discontinuation of medication, although less-strict weight-loss goals are suggested for those with type 2 diabetes [2]. It is recommended that orlistat treatment is continued for as long as clinical benefit is evident, and this includes the prevention of weight regain after a period of weight loss, which may mean prescribing outside current license [88]. Given its mode of action, orlistat has the potential to lower fat-soluble vitamins (A, D, E and beta carotene), although studies suggest levels generally remain within reference ranges [90]. However, given the increasing recognition of a higher risk of micronutrient deficiencies in the obese, it seems prudent to advise a multivitamin and mineral supplement to cover 100% daily recommended values. This should be taken just before bedtime to optimise absorption.

In a meta-analysis of orlistat trials (using 120 mg at three mealtimes), a 2.7 kg greater loss was achieved using orlistat+diet compared to placebo+diet [90]. Beneficial effects on serum cholesterol and low-density lipoproteins (LDLs), independent of weight loss, have also been observed [92]. In the XENDOS trial, a four-year randomised placebo-controlled study in overweight individuals, some with impaired glucose tolerance, a 6.9% weight loss was still evident in the orlistat-treated group at the end of the 4-year period, compared to a 4.1% loss in the placebo group [93]. A 37% reduction in the conversion of impaired glucose tolerance to type 2 diabetes was also found.

Alli is the over-the-counter version of orlistat, containing 60 mg rather than the 120 mg in prescription orlistat. It can be used in those with BMI ≥28 kg/m² and should be taken for no longer than 6 months. If no weight loss occurs after 12 weeks, health-professional support is recommended. As with the prescription version of orlistat, it is essential that a comprehensive lifestyle programme is adopted, with sufficient support provided to help the patient change their eating and activity behaviour long-term. The outcomes of the 'real-world' use of this medication are awaited with interest.

Surgical treatment

Surgical treatment is the most effective strategy for the management of severe and complex obesity. In a systematic review of surgical treatment in patients with a BMI >35 kg/m² and obesity-related co-morbidities, excess weight loss ranged from 52.5 to 77% at 10 years post-surgery [94], and there seems to be good maintenance over time [95–97]. In a study comparing a surgically treated group with a BMI-matched non-surgically managed group, overall mortality was 29–40% lower in the surgical group, with a 49% lower CVD mortality and 60% lower mortality from cancer [97,98]. However, there was substantially higher mortality in the surgical group from non-disease-related causes such as suicide. The associated explanation is unknown, but it highlights the importance of a comprehensive baseline assessment of psychological state. In those recently diagnosed with type 2 diabetes, the likelihood of substantial improvements in glycaemic control is high, with one study suggesting remission of diabetes in 73% of surgically treated subjects versus 13% of those managed with lifestyle modification [99]. There is also evidence supporting the benefit of surgery to quality of life [96], social interaction and depression [100].

The success of surgery depends on carefully selecting individuals with severe and complex obesity who are likely to benefit from a surgical approach. This is a clinical challenge, but NICE suggests the following guidance [2]:

- They have a BMI of 40 kg/m² or more, or between 35 and 40 kg/m² and other significant disease (for example, type 2 diabetes, high blood pressure) that could be improved if they lost weight.
- All appropriate nonsurgical measures have failed to achieve or maintain adequate clinically beneficial weight loss for at least 6 months.
- They are receiving or will receive intensive specialist management.
- They are generally fit for anaesthesia and surgery.
- They commit to the need for long-term follow-up.

Consider surgery as a first-line option for adults with a BMI of more than 50 kg/m² in whom surgical intervention is considered appropriate; consider orlistat before surgery if the waiting time is long.

It is important to ensure that patients deemed eligible for bariatric surgery have received appropriate education and support on the lifestyle implications of the surgical procedure in question. Rarely do patients reach an 'ideal' weight following bariatric surgery and perceptions of target weights achievable need to be considered, together with the possibility of weight regain.

Conclusion

Evidence supports multicomponent interventions combining diet, physical activity and behaviour modification. Following stabilisation of eating, as well as improvements to the quality of the diet, the evidence supports low-fat diets, the 600 kcal deficit approach, meal replacements and, in carefully selected individuals, VLCDs. In patients with higher BMIs, particularly those with associated morbidity, pharmacotherapy and/or surgery may be helpful. However, even when adjunct treatments are used, the lifestyle component of overall management remains central, and ongoing education and support critical.

References

1. Shaw K, Gennat H, O'Rourke P, Del Mar C. Exercise for overweight and obesity. Cochrane Database of Systematic Reviews; 2006. Report No.: Issue 4. Art No.: CD003817.DO1:10.1002/14651858CD003817.pub3.
2. National Institute for Clinical Excellence. Obesity: Guidance on the Prevention, Identification, Assessment and Management of Overweight and Obesity in Adults and Children. NICE; 2006.
3. Cho S, Dietrich M, Brown CJ, Clark CA, Block G. The effect of breakfast type on total daily energy intake and body mass index: results from the Third National Health and Nutrition Examination Survey (NHANES III). J Am Coll Nutr 2003 Aug;22[4]:296–302.

4. Ma Y, Bertone ER, Stanek EJ, 3rd, Reed GW, Hebert JR, Cohen NL, et al. Association between eating patterns and obesity in a free-living US adult population. Am J Epidemiol 2003 Jul 1;158[1]:85–92.

5. Song WO, Chun OK, Obayashi S, Cho S, Chung CE. Is consumption of breakfast associated with body mass index in US adults? J Am Diet Assoc 2005 Sep;105[9]:1373–82.

6. Wyatt HR, Grunwald GK, Mosca CL, Klem ML, Wing RR, Hill JO. Long-term weight loss and breakfast in subjects in the National Weight Control Registry. Obes Res 2002 Feb;10[2]:78–82.

7. Martin A, Normand S, Sothier M, Peyrat J, Louche-Pelissier C, Laville M. Is advice for breakfast consumption justified? Results from a short-term dietary and metabolic experiment in young healthy men. Br J Nutr 2000 Sep;84[3]:337–44.

8. Schlundt DG, Hill JO, Sbrocco T, Pope-Cordle J, Sharp T. The role of breakfast in the treatment of obesity: a randomized clinical trial. Am J Clin Nutr 1992 Mar;55[3]:645–51.

9. American Dietetic Association. Adult Weight Management Evidence Based Nutrition Practice Guideline; cited 2011 Jun 13). Available from: www.adaevidencelibrary.com.

10. Basdevant A, Craplet C, Guy-Grand B. Snacking patterns in obese French women. Appetite 1993 Aug;21[1]:17–23.

11. Drummond SE, Crombie NE, Cursiter MC, Kirk TR. Evidence that eating frequency is inversely related to body weight status in male, but not female, non-obese adults reporting valid dietary intakes. Int J Obes Relat Metab Disord 1998 Feb;22[2]:105–12.

12. Jonnalagadda SS, Harnack L, Hai Liu R, McKeown N, Seal C, Liu S, et al. Putting the whole grain puzzle together: health benefits associated with whole grains – summary of American Society for Nutrition 2010 satellite symposium. J Nutr 2011 May; 141[5]:1011S–22S.

13. Hung HC, Joshipura KJ, Jiang R, Hu FB, Hunter D, Smith-Warner SA, et al. Fruit and vegetable intake and risk of major chronic disease. J Natl Cancer Inst 2004 Nov 3;96[21]:1577–84.

14. Kris-Etherton PM, Harris WS, Appel LJ. Fish consumption, fish oil, omega-3 fatty acids, and cardiovascular disease. Circulation 2002 Nov 19;106[21]:2747–57.

15. Ernst B, Thurnheer M, Schmid SM, Schultes B. Evidence for the necessity to systematically assess micronutrient status prior to bariatric surgery. Obes Surg 2009 Jan;19[1]:66–73.

16. Flancbaum L, Belsley S, Drake V, Colarusso T, Tayler E. Preoperative nutritional status of patients undergoing Roux-en-Y gastric bypass for morbid obesity. J Gastrointest Surg 2006 Jul–Aug;10[7]:1033–7.

17. Astrup A, Grunwald GK, Melanson EL, Saris WH, Hill JO. The role of low-fat diets in body weight control: a meta-analysis of ad libitum dietary intervention studies. Int J Obes Relat Metab Disord 2000 Dec;24[12]:1545–52.

18. Frost G, Masters K, King C, Kelly M, Hasan U, Heavens S, et al. A new method of energy prescription to improve weight loss. J Hum Nutr Dietet 1991;4:369–73.

19. Avenell A, Broom J, Brown J, Poobalan A, Ancott L, Stearns S. Systematic Review of the Long-Term Effects and Economic Consequences of Treatments for Obesity and Implications for Health Improvements. Winchester, UK: Helath Technology Assessment; 2004.

20. Department of Health. Dietary Reference Values for Food, Energy and Nutrients for the United Kingdom. London: HMSO; 1991.

21. Heymsfield SB, van Mierlo CA, van der Knaap HC, Heo M, Frier HI. Weight management using a meal replacement strategy: meta and pooling analysis from six studies. Int J Obes Relat Metab Disord 2003 May;27[5]:537–49.

22. American Dietetic Association. Effectiveness in terms of client adherance and weight loss and maintenance of meal replacements. ADA; 2006.

23. STAN C. Standard for Formula Foods for Use in Very Low Energy Diets for Weight Reduction; 1995. Report No.: 203.

24. SCOOP. Reports on Tasks for Scientific Cooperation. Collection of Data on Products Intended for Use in Very Low Calorie Diets. Report of Events Participating in Task; 2002 Mar 7.

25. Pekkarinen T, Takala I, Mustajoki P. Two year maintenance of weight loss after a VLCD and behavioural therapy for obesity: correlation to the scores of questionnaires measuring eating behaviour. Int J Obes Relat Metab Disord 1996 Apr;20[4]: 332–7.

26. Foster-Powell K, Holt SH, Brand-Miller JC. International table of glycemic index and glycemic load values: 2002. Am J Clin Nutr 2002 Jul;76[1]:5–56.

27. Atkinson F, McMillan-Price J, Petocz P, Brand-Millar J. Physiological validation of the concept of glycaemic load in mixed meals over 10 hours in overweight females. Asia Pac J Clin Nutr 2004;13[suppl.]:S42.

28. Brand-Millar J, Thomas M, Swan V, Ahmad Z, Petocz P, Colagiuri S. Physiological validation of the concept of glyceamic load in lean young adults. J Nutr 2003;133: 2728–32.

29. Brand-Miller JC, Holt SH, Pawlak D, Mcmillan J. Glycemic index and obesity. Am J Clin Nutr 2002;76[suppl.]:281 S–285 S.

30. Brand-Millar J. Glycaemic index and body weight. Am J Clin Nutr 2005;81:722–3.

31. Sloth B, Krog-Mikkelsen I, Flint A, Tetans I, Astrup A, Raben A. Reply to J Brand Miller. Am J Clin Nutr 2005;81:723.

32. Sloth B, Astrup A. Low glycemic index diets and body weight. Int J Obes (Lond) 2006 Dec;30[Suppl. 3]:S47–51.

33. Thomas D, Elliot E, Baur L. Low glycaemic index or low glycaemic load diets for over-weight and obesity. Cochrane Database of Systematic Reviews; 2007.

34. Larsen TM, Dalskov S-M, van Baak M, Jebb SA, Papadaki A, Pfeiffer AFH, Martinez JA, Handjieva-Darlenska T, Kunešová M, Pihlsgård M, Stender S, Holst C, Saris WHM, Astrup A for the Diet, Obesity, and Genes (Diogenes) Project. Diets with high or low protein content and glycemic index for weight-loss maintenance. N Engl J Med 2010;363:2102–2113.

35. Lean ME, Lara J. Is Atkins dead (again)? Nutr Metab Cardiovasc Dis 2004 Apr;14[2]:61–5.

36. Harper A, Astrup A. Can we advise our obese patients to follow the Atkins diet? Obes Rev 2004 May;5[2]:93–4.

37. Freedman M, King J, Kennedy E. Popular diets: a scientific review. Obes Res 2001; Suppl. 1:1S–40S.

38. Due A, Toubro S, Skov AR, Astrup A. Effect of normal-fat diets, either medium or high in protein, on body weight in overweight subjects: a randomised 1-year trial. Int J Obes Relat Metab Disord 2004;28:1283–90.

39. Roberts DC. Quick weight loss: sorting fad from fact. Med J Aust 2001 Dec 3–17;175[11–12]:637–40.

40. Fox KR, Page A. The physical activity approach to the treatment of overweight and obesity. In: Kopelman PG, editor. Management of Obesity and Related Disorders. London: Martin Dunitz; 2001.

41. Douketis JD, Macie C, Thabane L, Williamson DF. Systematic review of long-term weight loss studies in obese adults: clinical significance and applicability to clinical practice. Int J Obes (Lond) 2005 Oct;29[10]:1153–67.

42. McTigue KM, Harris R, Hemphill B, Lux L, Sutton S, Bunton AJ, et al. Screening and interventions for obesity in adults: summary of the evidence for the US Preventive Services Task Force. Ann Intern Med 2003 Dec 2;139[11]:933–49.

43. Curioni CC, Lourenco PM. Long-term weight loss after diet and exercise: a systematic review. Int J Obes (Lond) 2005 Oct;29[10]:1168–74.

44. US Department of Health and Human Services. Physical Activity and Health: A Report of the Surgeon General. Atlanta, GA: US Department of Health and Human Services, Public Health Service, CDC, National Center for Chronic Disease Prevention and Health Promotion; 1996.

45. Klem ML, Wing RR, McGuire MT, Seagle HM, Hill JO. A descriptive study of individuals successful at long-term maintenance of substantial weight loss. Am J Clin Nutr 1997 Aug;66[2]:239–46.

46. Leitzmann MF, Park Y, Blair A, Ballard-Barbash R, Mouw T, Hollenbeck AR, et al. Physical activity recommendations and decreased risk of mortality. Arch Intern Med 2007 Dec 10;167[22]:2453–60.

47. Foreyt JP, Brunner RL, Goodrick GK, St Jeor ST, Miller GD. Psychological correlates of reported physical activity in normal-weight and obese adults: the Reno diet-heart study. Int J Obes Relat Metab Disord 1995 Oct;19[Suppl. 4]:S69–72.

48. Tremblay A, Despres JP, Leblanc C, Craig CL, Ferris B, Stephens T, et al. Effect of intensity of physical activity on body fatness and fat distribution. Am J Clin Nutr 1990 Feb;51[2]:153–7.

49. Williamson DF, Madans J, Anda RF, Kleinman JC, Kahn HS, Byers T. Recreational physical activity and ten-year weight change in a US national cohort. Int J Obes Relat Metab Disord 1993 May;17[5]:279–86.

50. Paffenbarger RS, Jr, Wing AL, Hyde RT, Jung DL. Physical activity and incidence of hypertension in college alumni. Am J Epidemiol 1983 Mar;117[3]:245–57.

51. Sandvik L, Erikssen J, Thaulow E, Erikssen G, Mundal R, Rodahl K. Physical fitness as a predictor of mortality among healthy, middle-aged Norwegian men. N Engl J Med 1993 Feb 25;328[8]:533–7.

52. Ross R, Dagnone D, Jones PJ, Smith H, Paddags A, Hudson R, et al. Reduction in obesity and related co-morbid conditions after diet-induced weight loss or exercise-induced weight loss in men. A randomized, controlled trial. Ann Intern Med 2000 Jul 18;133[2]:92–103.

53. Ivy JL, Zderic TW, Fogt DL. Prevention and treatment of non-insulin-dependent diabetes mellitus. Exerc Sport Sci Rev 1999;27:1–35.

54. Taylor AH, Fox KR. Effectiveness of a primary care exercise referral intervention for changing physical self-perceptions over 9 months. Health Psychol 2005 Jan; 24 [1]:11–21.

55. Penedo FJ, Dahn JR. Exercise and well-being: a review of mental and physical health benefits associated with physical activity. Curr Opin Psychiatry 2005 Mar;18[2]: 189–93.

56. Fox K. Self esteem, self perception and exercise. International Journal of Sport Psychology 2000;31:228–40.

57. Wadden TA, Foster GD, Letizia KA, Mullen JL. Long-term effects of dieting on resting metabolic rate in obese outpatients. JAMA 1990 Aug 8;264[6]:707–11.

58. King AC, Tribble DL. The role of exercise in weight regulation in nonathletes. Sports Med 1991 May;11[5]:331–49.

59. National Taskforce on the Prevention and Treatment of Obesity. Overweight, obesity and health risk. Arch Intern Med 2000;160:898–904.

60. Physical Activity Guidelines Advisory Committee Report to the Secretary of Health and Human Services US Department of Health and Human Services Web site; 2008.

61. BHF National Centre for Physical Activity and Health. Physical Activity Guidelines in the UK: Review and Recommendations. Loughborough University; 2010.

62. Department of Health. A Report on Physical Activity for Health from the Four Home Countries; 2011.

63. Saris WH, Blair SN, van Baak MA, Eaton SB, Davies PS, Di Pietro L, et al. How much physical activity is enough to prevent unhealthy weight gain? Outcome of the IASO 1st Stock Conference and consensus statement. Obes Rev 2003 May;4[2]:101–14.

64. Jeffery RW, Wing RR, Sherwood NE, Tate DF. Physical activity and weight loss: does prescribing higher physical activity goals improve outcome? Am J Clin Nutr 2003 Oct;78[4]:684–9.

65. Dunn AL, Marcus BH, Kampert JB, Garcia ME, Kohl HW, 3rd, Blair SN. Comparison of lifestyle and structured interventions to increase physical activity and cardiorespiratory fitness: a randomized trial. JAMA 1999 Jan 27;281[4]:327–34.

66. Andersen RE, Wadden TA, Bartlett SJ, Zemel B, Verde TJ, Franckowiak SC. Effects of lifestyle activity vs structured aerobic exercise in obese women: a randomized trial. JAMA 1999 Jan 27;281[4]:335–40.

67. Williams NH, Hendry M, France B, Lewis R, Wilkinson C. Effectiveness of exercise-referral schemes to promote physical activity in adults: systematic review. Br J Gen Pract 2007 Dec;57[545]:979–86.

68. Norris SL, Zhang X, Avenell A, Gregg E, Bowman B, Serdula M, et al. Long-term effectiveness of lifestyle and behavioral weight loss interventions in adults with type 2 diabetes: a meta-analysis. Am J Med 2004 Nov 15;117[10]:762–74.

69. Miller W, Rollnick S. Motivational interviewing: preparing people to change. New York: Guilford Press; 2002.

70. Funnell MM, Anderson RM, Arnold MS, Barr PA, Donnelly M, Johnson PD, et al. Empowerment: an idea whose time has come in diabetes education. Diabetes Educ 1991 Jan–Feb;17[1]:37–41.

71. Anderson RM, Funnell MM. Patient empowerment: reflections on the challenge of fostering the adoption of a new paradigm. Patient Educ Couns 2005 May;57[2]:153–7.

72. Bensing J. Bridging the gap. The separate worlds of evidenced based medicine and patient centred medicine. Patient Educ Couns 2000;39:17–25.

73. Stewart M. Patient Centred Medicine, Transforming the Clinical Method. Sage; 1995.

74. Mulvihill C, Quigley R. The management of obesity and overweight: an analysis of a review of diet, physical activity and behavioural approaches. London: Health Development Agency; 2003.

75. Najavits LM, Weiss RD. Variations in therapist effectiveness in the treatment of patients with substance use disorders: an empirical review. Addiction 1994 Jun;89[6]:679–88.

76. Knight KM, Dornan T, Bundy C. The diabetes educator: trying hard, but must concentrate more on behaviour. Diabet Med 2006 May;23[5]:485–501.

77. Baker R, Kirschenbaum DS. Self-monitoring may be necessary for successful weight control. Behaviour Therapy 1993;24:377–94.

78. Boutelle KN, Kirschenbaum DS. Further support for consistent self-monitoring as a vital component of successful weight control. Obes Res 1998 May;6[3]:219–24.

79. Hill J, Wing R. The National Weight Control Registry. The Permante Journal 2003;7:34–7.

80. Rapoport L, Pearson D. Health behaviour change. In: Thomas B, editor. The Manual of Dietetic Practice. Oxford: Blackwell Science; 2007.

81. Foreyt JP, Paschali A. Behavior therapy. In: Kopelman P, editor. Management of Obesity and Related Disorders. London: Martin Dunitz; 2001.

82. Wing RR, Tate DF, Gorin AA, Raynor HA, Fava JL. A self-regulation program for maintenance of weight loss. N Engl J Med 2006 Oct 12;355[15]:1563–71.
83. Kayman S, Bruvold W, Stern JS. Maintenance and relapse after weight loss in women: behavioral aspects. Am J Clin Nutr 1990 Nov;52[5]:800–7.
84. Wadden T, Phelan S. Behavioural assessment of the obese patient. In: Wadden T, Stunkard A, editors. Handbook of Obesity Treatment. New York: The Guilford Press; 2002. pp. 186–226.
85. Brownell KD. Weight cycling. Am J Clin Nutr 1989 May;49[5 Suppl.]:937.
86. Kramer FM, Jeffery RW, Snell MK. Monetary incentives to improve follow-up data collection. Psychol Rep 1986 Jun;58[3]:739–42.
87. Wadden TA, Berkowitz RI, Womble LG, Sarwer DB, Phelan S, Cato RK, et al. Randomized trial of lifestyle modification and pharmacotherapy for obesity. N Engl J Med 2005 Nov 17;353[20]:2111–20.
88. Linne Y, Rooth P, Rossner S. Success rate of Orlistat in primary-care practice is limited by failure to follow prescribing recommendations: the referral letter content vs clinical reality. Int J Obes Relat Metab Disord 2003 Nov;27[11]:1434–5.
89. Scottish Intercollegiate Guidelines Network. Management of Obesity: A National Clinical Guideline. SIGN; 2010.
90. Hollander PA, Elbein SC, Hirsch IB, Kelley D, McGill J, Taylor T, et al. Role of orlistat in the treatment of obese patients with type 2 diabetes. A 1-year randomized double-blind study. Diabetes Care 1998 Aug;21[8]:1288–94.
91. Haddock CK, Poston WS, Dill PL, Foreyt JP, Ericsson M. Pharmacotherapy for obesity: a quantitative analysis of four decades of published randomized clinical trials. Int J Obes Relat Metab Disord 2002 Feb;26[2]:262–73.
92. Bray GA, Greenway FL. Current and potential drugs for treatment of obesity. Endocr Rev 1999 Dec;20[6]:805–75.
93. Torgerson JS, Hauptman J, Boldrin MN, Sjostrom L. XENical in the prevention of diabetes in obese subjects (XENDOS) study: a randomized study of orlistat as an adjunct to lifestyle changes for the prevention of type 2 diabetes in obese patients. Diabetes Care 2004 Jan;27[1]:155–61.
94. O'Brien PE, McPhail T, Chaston TB, Dixon JB. Systematic review of medium-term weight loss after bariatric operations. Obes Surg 2006 Aug;16[8]:1032–40.
95. Gunther K, Vollmuth J, Weissbach R, Hohenberger W, Husemann B, Horbach T. Weight reduction after an early version of the open gastric bypass for morbid obesity: results after 23 years. Obes Surg 2006 Mar;16[3]:288–96.
96. Velcu LM, Adolphine R, Mourelo R, Cottam DR, Angus LD. Weight loss, quality of life and employment status after Roux-en-Y gastric bypass: 5-year analysis. Surg Obes Relat Dis 2005 Jul–Aug;1[4]:413–6; disc. 7.
97. Sjostrom L, Narbro K, Sjostrom CD, Karason K, Larsson B, Wedel H, et al. Effects of bariatric surgery on mortality in Swedish obese subjects. N Engl J Med 2007 Aug 23;357[8]:741–52.
98. Adams TD, Gress RE, Smith SC, Halverson RC, Simper SC, Rosamond WD, et al. Long-term mortality after gastric bypass surgery. N Engl J Med 2007 Aug 23;357[8]:753–61.
99. Dixon JB, O'Brien PE, Playfair J, Chapman L, Schachter LM, Skinner S, et al. Adjustable gastric banding and conventional therapy for type 2 diabetes: a randomized controlled trial. JAMA 2008 Jan 23;299[3]:316–23.
100. Karlsson J, Taft C, Ryden A, Sjostrom L, Sullivan M. Ten-year trends in health-related quality of life after surgical and conventional treatment for severe obesity: the SOS intervention study. Int J Obes (Lond) 2007 Aug;31[8]:1248–61.

2 Practical Application

4 Preventing Overweight and Obesity

'Obesity is a chronic relapsing disease' [1].

Prevention of overweight and obesity

The prevention of obesity is complex as there are many factors which influence weight gain. Tackling the 'obesogenic environment' through multi-agency approaches needs to be a priority [2].

The obesogenic environment

This is defined as 'the total sum of influences in the environment on promoting obesity in individuals and populations' [2].

Practitioners will have opportunities to intervene to prevent weight gain at different stages of life:

Pre-conception and antenatal care

Up to 50% of pregnancies are likely to be unplanned [3], so all women of childbearing age need to be aware of the importance of a healthy diet. Nutritional interventions for women who are, or who plan to become, pregnant are likely to have the greatest effect if delivered before conception and during the first 12 weeks [3]. A healthy diet is important for both the baby and the mother throughout pregnancy and after the birth. Therefore, action should include providing women with information on the benefits of a healthy diet [4] (Resources 4 and 5).

The early years

There is an association between breastfeeding and reduced obesity in later childhood, suggesting some potential protective effect [5]. Ideally, anthropometric measurements should be tracked from an early age to ensure that length/height and weight progress within normal BMI centile ranges for infancy and childhood. When BMI exceeds the 91st centile, it is advisable to begin to consider healthy eating, portion control and activity measures to prevent further weight gain in childhood. Prevention of overweight and obesity in childhood should address lifestyle within family and social settings [6] (Resource 6).

As life goes by

In adulthood, weight gain can occur at various stages and often coincides with life events such as leaving home, change in employment, moving in with a partner or retirement. In addition, certain groups/individuals are more at risk of becoming overweight, for example where one or both parents are overweight, certain ethnic groups, those with learning disabilities and those on low income.

Encouraging adults to maintain a healthy weight is prudent in terms of health promotion and disease prevention. Medical notes should track BMI changes from early adulthood, helping to highlight any significant increase in BMI, which can then be addressed through healthy eating and activity measures to prevent further weight gain.

Health professionals have an opportunity to discuss weight, diet and activity with people at times when weight gain is more likely, such as during and after pregnancy, the menopause and after smoking cessation [6]. Periods of inactivity due to illness or injury may also precipitate weight gain.

On average, adults gain 0.5–1.5 lb (0.2–0.7 kg) per year [7]. As life goes by, this can add up to a significant weight gain, resulting in overweight or obesity. Many people do not weigh themselves regularly and only become aware of a weight increase when their clothes feel tight, or when it is highlighted in a medical check-up.

Facts

An additional 100 calories per day = 10 lb (4.5 kg) per year gained
1 extra slice of bread = 100 calories
1 mile of brisk walking = 100 calories

Encouraging people to prevent weight gain is a crucial element in the prevention of overweight and obesity. Simple steps can help prevent weight gain being the inevitable consequence of ageing. To help prevent weight gain, practitioners can:

- Encourage activity and reduce sedentary behaviours, e.g. less TV and screen time.
- Encourage people to eat healthily and become more aware of what they eat.
- Encourage regular weight checks [8].

It has been shown that most people underestimate their food intake [9] and overestimate their levels of activity [10].

Medications

Certain medications are known to have an adverse effect on weight (see Chapter 1 and Appendix 6) and weight-management measures should be discussed with patients who are prescribed medications associated with weight gain [11].

What to do?

Look for changes in weight as part of routine health checks:

Weight **decrease** may be an indicator of other health problems – **explore**

Practitioner: *'Were you aware that your weight has dropped since your last check-up?'*

Weight remains **steady** (1–2 kg) within normal BMI range – **affirm**

Practitioner: *'It's good to see that your weight remains within the healthy range. Keeping your weight stable is really helpful in reducing your chances of developing various conditions, like diabetes.'*

Weight has **increased** by >3 kg (even when within normal BMI range) – **discuss**

Practitioner: *'Were you aware that your weight has increased since your last check-up?'*
Patient: *'No!'*
Practitioner: *'Well, you are still within the normal range so it is not a health concern at the moment. The reason I mention it is that many people who become overweight wish they had addressed it before it became a problem.'*
Patient: *'I guess that makes sense. Do you think I should go on a diet?'*
Practitioner: *'No, but it is worth looking at what has changed recently in relation to your eating and/or activity.'*
Patient: *'Nothing, really. I suppose I did change jobs 6 months ago and of course I am driving more and maybe I'm eating at different times…'*
Practitioner: *'A change in routine can often affect weight. A decrease in activity seems to make a big difference as well as what you eat.'*
Patient: *'I have been thinking about getting more exercise – I don't want to become unfit and I do feel sluggish if I spend most of the day behind the wheel and in meetings.'*
Practitioner: *'I guess it is a case of finding something that you enjoy and that fits in.'*
Patient: *'Yep, I'm on the case!'*
Practitioner: *'What about the food side of things?'*
Patient: *'Not so good, I have picked up some really bad habits! I need to get back to eating healthy food. I know it's the snacks that I need to tackle!'*
Practitioner: *'You are sounding very determined! I have a **leaflet** here that you might like to read through. It contains some very useful tips that you may find helpful.'* [Resource 7]
Patient: *'Yes, I will have a read – I certainly don't want my weight to creep up any further!'*

There are a number of reasons why patients may not be interested in addressing their weight at the time of the consultation and it is important that their choice not to act is respected.

If the response is negative

Example of discussion

Patient: '*I know I have put on a bit of weight but to be honest, I haven't got time to think about it at the moment.*'

Practitioner: '*It sounds like you are really busy and don't have time to think about your weight just now. Would you like to take this leaflet* [Resource 8], *and you can read about it in your own time? It explains why we are encouraging everyone to be conscious of their weight in relation to overall health.*'

Patient: '*OK.*'

Practitioner: '*If you want to discuss this again at any time, pop back and see me.*'

Support materials

Resource 8 highlights the importance of being a healthy weight. In one study, Lally and colleagues [12] developed an intervention which produced clinically significant weight loss. Participants were given a leaflet on habit formation and simple eating and activity behaviours to achieve negative energy balance, along with self-monitoring checklists. The leaflet describes ten top tips for weight loss (outlined below) and is now available through Cancer Research UK (Resource 7). It has potential use for those requiring modest weight loss or wishing to prevent weight gain.

Other useful resources

Change 4 Life resources are useful for family-based approaches (Resource 6). For pre-conception and pregnancy, Resources 4 and 5 are recommended. Resource 9 is also useful for those who want guidance on how to lose weight.

Ten top tips for weight loss [12]

1 **Keep to your meal routine**
   Try to eat at roughly the same times each day, whether this is two or five times a day.

2 **Go reduced-fat**
   Choose reduced-fat foods (e.g. dairy foods, spreads, salad dressings) where you can. Use high-fat foods (e.g. butter and oils) sparingly, if at all.

3 **Walk off the weight**
   Walk 10 000 steps (equivalent to 60–90 minutes' moderate activity) each day. You can use a pedometer to help count the steps.

4 **Pack a healthy snack**
   If you snack, choose a healthy option such as fresh fruit or low-calorie yogurts instead of chocolate or crisps.

5 **Learn the labels**
   Be careful about food claims. Check the fat and sugar content on food labels when shopping and preparing food.

6 **Caution with your portions**
   Do not heap food on your plate (except vegetables). Think twice before having second helpings.

7 **Up on your feet**
   Break up your sitting time. Stand up for 10 minutes out of every hour.

8 **Think about your drinks**
   Choose water or sugar-free squashes. Unsweetened fruit juice contains natural sugar so limit it to one glass a day (200 ml/one-third pint). Alcohol is high in calories; limit it to one unit a day for women and two for men.

9 **Focus on your food**
   Slow down. Do not eat on the go or while watching TV. Eat at a table if possible.

10 **Do not forget your five a day**
   Eat at least five portions of fruit and vegetables a day (400 g in total).

Conclusion

Maintaining a healthy weight throughout life is the ideal. Unfortunately, today's environment makes this very challenging for many people. Practitioners need to be aware of how easily weight gain can occur, especially in susceptible individuals. Steps to prevent early weight gain progressing to overweight and then obesity should be addressed at the earliest opportunity.

Reflective exercise: case study

A 35-year-old female attends a routine appointment for renewal of a pill prescription. She is wearing a track suit and has just come from an exercise class. Height: 168 cm.

	Weight history	BMI
Age 25 years:	58 kg	20.5
Age 30 years:	65 kg	23.0
Age 35 years:	70 kg	24.8

1 Would you discuss weight with this person?
2 If yes, what are your reasons and what might you say?
3 If no, what are your reasons?
4 Where is this lady's weight likely to be in 5 or 10 years' time?

References

1. Bray GA. Obesity is a chronic, relapsing neurochemical disease. Int J Obes Relat Metab Disord 2004 Jan;28[1]:34–8.
2. Butland B, Jebb S, Kopelman P. Tackling Obesities: Future Choices – Project Report. London: Foresight Programme of the Government Office for Science; 2007.
3. National Institute for Clinical Excellence. Improving the Nutrition of Pregnant and Breastfeeding Mothers and Children in Low-income Households. NICE Public Health Guidance 11. NICE; 2008.

4. National Institute for Clinical Excellence. Dietary Interventions and Physical Activity Interventions for Weight Management Before, During and After Pregnancy. NICE Public Health Guidance 27. NICE; 2010.

5. Arenz S, Ruckerl R, Koletzko B, von Kries R. Breast-feeding and childhood obesity – a systematic review. Int J Obes Relat Metab Disord 2004 Oct;28[10]:1247–56.

6. National Institute for Clinical Excellence. Obesity: Guidance on the Prevention, Identification, Assessment and Management of Overweight and Obesity in Adults and Children. NICE; 2006.

7. Yanovski JA, Yanovski SZ, Sovik KN, Nguyen TT, O'Neil PM, Sebring NG. A prospective study of holiday weight gain. N Engl J Med 2000 Mar 23;342[12]:861–7.

8. McGuire MT, Wing RR, Klem ML, Hill JO. Behavioral strategies of individuals who have maintained long-term weight losses. Obes Res 1999 Jul;7[4]:334–41.

9. Wansink B, Chandon P. Meal size, not body size, explains errors in estimating the calorie content of meals. Ann Intern Med 2006 Sep 5;145[5]:326–32.

10. Sallis JF, Haskell WL, Wood PD, Fortmann SP, Rogers T, Blair SN, et al. Physical activity assessment methodology in the Five-City Project. Am J Epidemiol 1985 Jan;121[1]:91–106.

11. Scottish Intercollegiate Guidelines Network. Obesity in Scotland 2010. A National Guideline for Use in Scotland. Edinburgh: SIGN; 2010.

12. Lally P, Chipperfield A, Wardle J. Healthy habits: efficacy of simple advice on weight control based on a habit-formation model. Int J Obes (Lond) 2008 Apr;32[4]:700–7.

5 Providing A Person-centred Weight-management Service

'I've learned that people will forget what you said, people will forget what you did, but people will never forget how you made them feel.'

Maya Angelou

Integrating a behavioural approach

Working in a person-centred way

When working with people to prevent or manage overweight and obesity, health practitioners should follow the principles of person-centred care [1], which consists of the following six components [2]:

1 Exploring the disease and the experience
2 Understanding the whole person
3 Finding common ground
4 Incorporating prevention and health promotion
5 Enhancing the helper–patient relationship
6 Being realistic.

These components fit very comfortably into weight-management interventions. Being person-centred is fundamental to **a behavioural approach** and including **behaviour-change strategies** improves outcomes achieved in weight-management programmes [1]. Good communication skills are essential and any behavioural intervention should be delivered by an appropriately trained professional [1].

Practitioners often struggle to truly integrate a behavioural approach in weight management, which may partly relate to confusion over its meaning and poor confidence in the skills which underpin this approach. A behavioural approach is both **directive** and **patient-centred**, and a **guiding** style can help combine both aspects [3]. In practice, this means a practitioner guides and supports the patient in the decision-making process. This includes whether it is the right time to start a programme and whether the patient feels able to commit to the necessary long-term

Weight Management: A Practitioner's Guide, First Edition. Dympna Pearson and Clare Grace.
© 2012 Dympna Pearson and Clare Grace. Published 2012 by Blackwell Publishing Ltd.

eating and activity changes. The practitioner guides the patient towards finding solutions that will work best for them by sharing ideas and expertise.

When practitioners consider a behavioural approach, they often think about tools and strategies they can use to get people to change. Although there are a number of useful tools and strategies, a behavioural approach is much more than this. It relies heavily on the spirit of the approach, working in a collaborative manner and adhering to the core conditions of a person-centred approach, empathy, genuineness and acceptance. The helping relationship is paramount as it underpins any behavioural strategy, and it should develop as the intervention progresses.

How to integrate a behavioural approach in practice?

Consider the patient experience

A helpful way to think about integrating a behavioural approach is to consider what the experience might be like from the patient's perspective. When providing weight-management services, think how the patient might feel walking into new surroundings. Ensure that they are made to feel welcome by all staff and that the surroundings are appropriate:

- Reading materials and educational posters should be weight-sensitive, i.e. not all 'super-skinny models'.
- Sturdy chairs (without arms) should be provided.
- Large blood-pressure cuffs need to be available.
- Adequate scales (weighing up to 250 kg) should be available (Appendix 1).
- All equipment should be checked regularly for accuracy.
- Ensure that all measurements are taken in a private area.

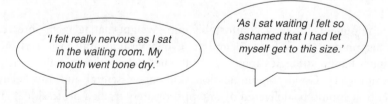

'I felt really nervous as I sat in the waiting room. My mouth went bone dry.'

'As I sat waiting I felt so ashamed that I had let myself get to this size.'

Consider which terminology to use

Many patients dislike being referred to as 'obese'. Although it is used as a medical term, if it causes offence, it may damage the helping relationship. 'Weight' is a more neutral term which is less likely to cause upset [4].

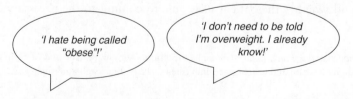

'I hate being called "obese"!'

'I don't need to be told I'm overweight. I already know!'

Listen empathically and try to understand what it is like for the patient

Weight management can be challenging and, at times, frustrating for the patient, and this can hinder progress. Listening is very powerful. It helps the patient to feel understood and it clarifies their story. When a helper fails to listen, the patient may be discouraged, the wrong issue may be discussed or a strategy may be proposed prematurely [4]. Listen with empathy when patients describe how difficult they find managing their weight.

Be mindful of how difficult it can be to change eating and activity habits

Breaking old habits and forming new habits requires:

- Effort
- Energy
- Commitment
- Focus
- Time
- Sacrifice
- Lots of practice of new skills/habits
- And much more!

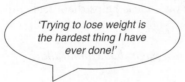

'Trying to lose weight is the hardest thing I have ever done!'

Affirm every effort: affirmations help to build people's confidence in their ability to change. Patients respond well to any words of encouragement, such as 'You have managed really well!', but to be effective, affirmations must always be genuine. Pay particular attention to tone of voice to avoid sounding patronising.

Consider motivation at the outset and throughout the programme/intervention

Patients should have the opportunity to make informed decisions about their care and treatment, in partnership with their health professionals [1]. It is not for the practitioner to decide whether someone is 'ready' or not. There needs to be a joint discussion about whether the patient feels willing and able, at this point in time, to make the necessary commitment. When using motivational tools, good interpersonal skills are essential as they can strongly influence motivation and change [5].

Most guidelines recommend 'assessing motivation' or 'assessing readiness to change' before commencing a weight-management intervention [1,6]. Motivation is also required throughout the whole process of losing weight *and* in the prevention of weight regain. As motivation fluctuates over time, it should be revisited on a regular basis throughout the intervention, not just at the beginning.

Successful weight-management involves sustained changes to eating and activity behaviours, which are notoriously difficult and require high levels of commitment. It is essential to check throughout the treatment period whether weight management continues to be a priority for the individual. If the patient is not fully engaged in the process, repeated failed attempts can damage their belief that weight loss is possible.

Motivation

Motivational interviewing is a collaborative conversation style for strengthening a person's own motivation and commitment to change [7]

Importance and **Confidence** are considered to be the key constructs of motivation: if a change feels important to you, and you have the confidence to achieve it, you will feel more **ready** to have a go, and you are more likely to succeed [8]. Conversations that **explore** importance and confidence can greatly influence motivation.

See examples of exploring motivation in the section on 'Exploring Whether This Is the Right Time to Begin', later in this chapter.

Resist the urge to 'fix it'

Practitioners often find it difficult to resist the urge to tell people what to do or to provide solutions. This probably comes from a strong desire to be helpful but it can have the opposite effect of increasing resistance to change. Encouraging patients to explore their own ideas helps them feel empowered to find their own solutions:

> 'I wonder what ideas you might have about that.'

Remember to value any suggestions they make. Suggestions can, and should, be made by the practitioner but they must be put forward in a respectful manner. Making uninvited suggestions is likely to be met with the 'Yes, but...' response. Respecting patient autonomy (acknowledging that the patient has the right to make decisions regarding their own behaviour) is a key principle of working in a behavioural way. Always **ask permission** to put forward your suggestions; for example:

> 'Would you like me to make some suggestions?'

Try to avoid:

> 'Do you think you can...?'
> 'What you need to do is...'
> 'I think you should...' or 'If I were you...'

The natural response to these suggestions is for the patient to object or disagree, which may sound like 'excuses'. Such a 'fix it' approach is unlikely to lead to sustained behaviour change on the part of the patient and is likely to leave the practitioner feeling frustrated.

Be optimistic, but realistic

If someone has failed to lose weight previously and feels hopeless, this may begin to influence the practitioner's attitude to the likelihood of success. If a practitioner believes a patient is unlikely to change, there is a high chance that this negative attitude will be transmitted to the patient.

We have to believe a patient can do it; our own belief in the person's ability to change can become a self-fulfilling prophecy [6]. If we believe a patient can change, we will act in a way that increases the likelihood the patient will do so. It is important to convey optimism in their ability to succeed. This needs to be expressed as being quietly confident rather than as a 'gung-ho' style of optimism. '*You have some good ideas there, which sound as if they would work for you,*' is likely to be more effective *than, 'Of course you can do it!'*

Helping individuals to set realistic goals can contribute to a sense of optimism: '*Half a stone – I can manage that.*'

In this book, we have tried to integrate the principles of a behavioural approach in a very practical way, where possible.

Consider this

A person with high blood pressure and a BMI of 35 attends for an initial weight-management consultation.

- What thoughts might be going through their mind?
- How are they feeling?
- What concerns might they have?
- What thoughts are going through your mind?
- What can you do to ensure that it is a positive experience?

Identifying overweight and obesity

Body mass index (BMI) is the recommended measure for identifying overweight and obesity. It requires both height (Appendix 2 and Resource 10) and weight (Appendix 3 and Resource 11) measures to be undertaken. Appendix 4 provides guidance on how to calculate BMI from height and weight.

The Department of Health has published Local Delivery Plans which require the NHS to return local data on BMI levels [9]. These provide information on the local and national incidence of obesity.

Interpreting BMI

The degree of overweight or obesity in adults should be defined as in Table 5.1 [1].

Waist circumference may be used, in addition to BMI, to refine the risk assessment of obesity-related co-morbidities in those with a BMI of less than $35 \, kg/m^2$ (Table 5.2) [1,5].

Currently, there is no global agreement on waist cut-off points for different ethnic groups.

Table 5.1   Classification of overweight/obesity in adults (Nice 2006 [1])

Classification	BMI (kg/m^2)
Healthy weight	18.5–24.9
Overweight	25–29.9
Obesity I	30–34.9
Obesity II	35–39.9
Obesity III	40 or more

Note: BMI should be interpreted with caution as it is not a direct measure of adiposity (amount of body fat). Take care when interpreting BMI in muscular individuals [1] or certain ethnic groups. Although not yet validated, lower BMI cut-off points may be appropriate for those of South Asian, Chinese and Japanese origin, where individuals are considered overweight at BMI >23 kg/m^2 and obese at BMI >27.5 kg/m^2 [5].

Table 5.2   Waist circumference thresholds used to assess health risks in the general population (Nice 2006 [1])

Risk level	Male	Female
Increased risk	94 cm (37 inches) or more	80 cm (31 inches) or more
Greatly increased risk	102 cm (40 inches) or more	88 cm (35 inches) or more

Although measuring waist circumference superficially seems an easy procedure, it can be affected by a number of factors, including patient movement or position, poor positioning of the measuring tape and the amount of tape tension applied by the practitioner. Changes in these factors can affect measurement reliability. It is also important to be mindful that for some individuals, measurement of waist may feel more intrusive than of weight, and it should always be undertaken in a skilled and sensitive manner. See Appendix 5 and Resource 12 for guidance on how to measure waist circumference.

Planning weight-management interventions in your setting

Aiming for a coordinated and structured approach

A structured and coordinated approach is essential for effective weight management. This should include a patient pathway and accompanying protocols which clearly define the roles and responsibilities of practitioners [10]. There are many pathways in existence and these are intended to help services and individual practitioners deliver structured and cohesive weight-management interventions [5,11,12]. Local services may wish to adapt what is already available to meet the needs of their local population. For this purpose, the Obesity Care Pathway Support Package produced by Public Health Action Support Team is a helpful guidance document [13].

It is recommended that any health professional involved in obesity treatment should have received specific training and attained relevant competencies [1,14]. It is also essential to evaluate the effectiveness of any intervention or service [1] (see Chapter 11).

The overweight population is heterogeneous, with wide variations in age, gender, cultural differences and degree of overweight. Although obesity is more prevalent in some communities, it is not exclusive to any one group. A wide range of interventions exist in health care services and the commercial sector, and from the patient's perspective, the quantity and quality of choices available can be confusing. Most overweight people will try a number of different approaches with varying success. Effective weight management needs to ensure that treatment options are tailored to meet the needs of the individual.

It is now clear that weight-management interventions need to be well designed and delivered in a structured way in order to optimise their effectiveness. Ad hoc interventions, such as one-off, intermittent or repeated advice to 'eat less and exercise more' are at best an extravagant waste of limited resources, and at worst risk damaging the patient's belief in their ability to successfully manage their weight (see Chapter 10 for more on how to manage contacts when time is limited).

Deciding on the duration and frequency of appointments

Duration of treatment

The duration of weight-loss programmes varies hugely, although current practice favours a weight-loss phase of 3–6 months, aiming for 5–10% weight-loss outcome. In some cases, treatment may need to continue for up to 1 year or longer. Much will depend on the degree of obesity and the available resources. Some guidelines suggest the priority after 6 months should be weight maintenance achieved through sustained changes in physical activity and eating behaviours. After a period of weight maintenance, further weight loss can be considered [15].

Despite the well-documented success of weight-loss programmes, treatment is typically followed by weight regain. Therefore, the maintenance of treatment effects may be the greatest challenge in long-term obesity management, and **continuous care** may be required [16]. Obesity is a chronic relapsing disease needing lifelong management [17].

Frequency of appointments/contact

'It really helped seeing the nurse each week.'

'Patients seem to lose motivation if the gaps between appointments are too long.'
(health care professional)

Evidence suggests higher-intensity input produces better outcomes, and regular support from health professionals is recognised as a central feature of comprehensive weight management [1,18]. The National Obesity Observatory recommends that interventions allow sufficient time for consultations, plan to provide repeat consultations and arrange frequent follow-up appointments [19]. NICE Guidance recommends that support should be determined by the person's needs and be responsive to change over time [1].

The Counterweight Programme [20] is an example of a successful primary-care intervention which offers frequent appointments. It is a cost-effective, evidence-based UK primary-care programme that during the research trial produced mean weight losses of 3 kg over 12 months and 2.3 kg at 24 months. Patients attend nine appointments in the first year and six intensive education sessions (10–30 minutes) in the first 3 months. Education resources and a choice of weight-loss plans are also available. Thereafter, quarterly reviews over 9 months are followed by an annual review.

How and when to begin conversations about weight

Practitioners need to use their clinical judgment as to **when** to measure weight and height and must be skilled in **raising the issue** of overweight.

Health care professionals need to consider *when* it is appropriate to measure BMI. For example:

- a new-patient check or health-screening consultation
- when weight is related to the presenting health problem (high blood pressure, joint pain, breathing difficulties, etc.)
- when records indicate that BMI has not been checked for some time.

NB It is also important to recognise situations where raising the issue of weight is NOT appropriate, such as:

- when the person presents with an urgent medical problem
- when the person is clearly unwell
- when weight has already been discussed recently and received a negative response
- when the person has a serious ongoing medical problem that will not be helped by weight loss.

Raising the issue of weight is a sensitive topic for affected individuals and practitioners [14]. Overweight people may feel self-conscious or embarrassed about their weight or may have experienced negative attitudes and weight bias from health care professionals (see Chapter 2).

Practitioners often have concerns about raising the issue and discussing weight. These include:

- concerns about damaging the helping relationship
- fears of causing embarrassment or upset

- concerns that it feels like a personal comment
- fears of a defensive response
- concerns over their own weight and/or body image
- concerns about how to respond to comments about their own weight.

Practitioners with concerns about their own body image need to consider what impact these may have during a weight-management intervention. Self-help books can be a useful source of support (Resources 13 and 14), or it may be appropriate to seek help if one's own concerns about body image are negatively impacting on the helping relationship.

Many patients are unaware of the extent of their weight problem. Weight is an important health issue with serious health implications and it cannot be ignored. However, it needs to be raised in a way that is helpful, sensitive and supportive.

Examples of raising the issue

As part of a new patient check '*As part of the medical check we offer to all new patients, we include blood pressure, blood tests and weight checks. Is it OK with you if we do those measurements now?*'

OR

Linked to a health concern '*Weight can also affect … Would you like me to explain how weight affects your blood pressure/diabetes, etc.?*'

OR

When records indicate that BMI has not been checked for some time '*Your records show that you have not had a general health check for some time – would you like me to do that while you are here?*'

'*The nurse was lovely; she didn't make me feel embarrassed about my weight.*'

'*What a relief! I've always been afraid to bring up the subject of weight myself.*'

Responding to comments about your own weight

Sometimes patients may respond defensively when the issue of weight is raised and this can take the form of a comment about the practitioner's own weight. This is often an expression of the patient's frustration or fear of being judged, and the practitioner needs to convey understanding rather than reacting defensively or ignoring/skipping over the comment. References to the practitioner's weight are more likely to occur if the practitioner uses an advice-giving style where the patient feels they are being told what to do. In order to preserve the helping relationship, the response to comments about your own weight needs to be open, honest and nonjudgmental.

Example 1   (when the practitioner is overweight)

Patient: *'Perhaps you should take your own advice!'*
Practitioner: *'Can I check that because I am overweight you feel it is inappropriate for me to advise you in relation to your weight?'*
Patient: *'Well, yes.'*
Practitioner: *'I appreciate your concerns, and being overweight does make me very aware of how difficult it is to lose weight. However, I think it would be more helpful to focus on how we can find the best option for you. Are you happy to do that?'*
Patient: *'OK, what do you advise?'*
Practitioner: *'Well, there isn't one way that works for everyone, so what I'm hoping is that with my own experience, and that of working with others who struggle with their weight, along with your ideas on what works best for you, that we can come up with a solution that really works for you. How does that sound?'*

Avoid, *'I know what you mean!'* Conversations about the practitioner's weight can take the focus away from the patient.

Example 2 (when the practitioner is slim)

Patient: *'It's all very well for you – you don't have to worry about your weight.'*
Practitioner: *'Can I check that you feel I might not understand how difficult it is to lose weight?'*
Patient: *'Well, yes.'*
Practitioner: *'I appreciate your concerns and I hope that the experience I have gained of working with others who struggle with their weight has given me some insight into how difficult it is. What I'd like to suggest is that using that experience, along with your ideas of what will work for you, we will come up with the best solution for yourself. How does that sound?*
Patient: *'OK'*

Exploring whether this is the right time to begin

Exploring **motivation** and **readiness to change** – here the **importance** of losing weight is discussed.

Establishing initial interest

Practitioner: *'Is losing weight something you are **willing** to consider at the moment?'*
Patient: *'Yes, if it is starting to affect my health…'*
[Encourage the patient to discuss their reasons for wanting to lose weight – helps build and strengthen motivation]
Practitioner: *'You sound really up for it! There are a number of options but first it would be helpful to have a more complete picture – is it OK if I take some more measurements?*
Patient: *'OK.'*
Practitioner: *'That will help us to decide the best way forward.'*

1 If the response is positive, **record baseline data** and then move on to **explore options** and agree a way forward
2 If not, offer the opportunity to discuss this at a later date and provide an information leaflet, such as 'Why Weight Matters' (Resource 8). If possible, **record baseline data**

Example of recording weight and other baseline data

Invite the patient to be weighed: *'Can I ask you to step on the scales?'*
Request permission to take measurements: *'Is it OK if I check your waist measurement? Can I check your blood pressure now? Is it OK if I take some bloods?'*
Avoid: *'Now I want you to…', 'I need to…', 'Now we are going to…'*

Establish degree of obesity and assess risk factors by recording baseline data

• BMI (Appendices 2–4)
• waist measurement if BMI is less than 35 (Appendix 5)
• blood pressure
• fasting blood glucose
• lipid profile

Manage co-morbidities when they are identified – do not wait for the patient to lose weight [1]

More on motivation…

Is the patient really sure they have the time and commitment required?

Having raised the issue, it is important to check if the patient is **willing** to embark on a weight-management plan right now and if they feel **able** to commit to making the eating and activity changes required. At this point, the practitioner's role is to help the patient understand the level of commitment required to begin a weight-management programme.

Example of discussing options and the commitment required

Practitioner: *'Are you happy to think about what will help you lose weight?'*
Patient: *'Yes, definitely.'*
Practitioner: *'Now we have some measurements, we can look at which option is going to be best for you. Your results suggest that that the best treatment option for you would be* [refer to local pathway]*, how does that sound?'*
Patient: *'Can you tell me a bit more about what it involves?'*
[Explain what the service offers and the level of commitment required from the patient. Check whether the patient is happy with the recommended option.]
Practitioner: *'You sound keen to get started. Do you feel **able** to take this on **at this point in time**?'*
Patient: *'I think so, especially if I have some help with…'*

Discussing and agreeing a way forward

Once agreement to proceed has been established, and a treatment option has been chosen, it is essential that a thorough and an in-depth **assessment** is undertaken as a vital first step of the process.

Exploring treatment options

The level of intervention and the suitable treatment options will depend on the degree of obesity, existing co-morbidities and accompanying health risks. It is important to be familiar with local pathways and models of care, in order to match treatment options to the needs of the individual. The options include:

Lifestyle treatment

This will be relevant regardless of whether drugs or surgical treatment are considered. All weight-management programmes should include **behaviour change strategies** to:

- Improve eating behaviour and the quality of the patient's diet and reduce energy intake
- Increase the patient's physical activity levels and decrease inactivity

Lifestyle interventions can be provided in a variety of ways, including one-to-one interventions (the focus of this book) and group programmes. In most cases, with good support, patients can expect to lose 5–10% of their initial weight over 6 months. Some people may lose more, but it is unusual, so it is important to consider the limitations of what can be achieved with lifestyle treatments alone.

Group-based programmes

Group weight-management programmes offer another effective option for delivering lifestyle interventions and may be the preferred option for certain individuals. Some research suggests group treatment produces greater weight loss than individual therapy [21,22]. However, there is a need to develop a greater understanding of the characteristics of those who respond well to group treatment and determine what impact other factors, such as the skill level of the group leader, have on outcomes achieved. There is known to be variation in the types of group programme available in the 'real world', and given the importance of matching treatments to individual needs, there is likely to be a role for both individual and group interventions.

Potential benefits of group-based programmes

Group programmes can offer:

- Support from group leaders as well as peer support from other members.
- The potential to be more time-efficient, given practitioners can see larger numbers of patients in a specified period. However, an initial investment is needed to plan and prepare a group programme, which can be time-consuming. In addition, organisational time is required before and after each session.

What is available?

Within the NHS

Group programmes delivered in the NHS tend to vary in their design and duration, the length of each session, the topics included and the style of delivery. However, in most instances the core content covers information on diet, physical activity and behavioural strategies.

Commercial slimming clubs

There are numerous well-recognised commercial slimming clubs which overweight and obese people can pay to attend. Costs vary depending on the organisation and location but are about £5–6 (in 2011) for each weekly attendance, as well as an additional registration fee. Some organisations operate 'slimming on referral' schemes (usually 12 weeks) where patients are referred from primary care into a commercial slimming programme at either reduced or no cost to the patient.

Lay groups

Community weight-management groups are run either in community leisure services or by various volunteer organisations.

Setting up your own weight-management groups

The skills required to run group-based programmes differ from those needed for one-to-one interventions. It is important to ensure practitioners intending to set up new programmes have received training in group-facilitation skills and the use of behavioural skills in a group setting, and are competent to deliver evidence-based dietary and physical activity guidance.

If your service decides to set up and run a weight-management group, careful thought needs to be given to:

Planning

Consider:

- who will attend
  - o all overweight and obese individuals or those in certain BMI ranges; only male, only female or both genders; age ranges

- where the sessions will be held
  - o suitability, safety, convenience
- times and durations of sessions
- length of programme
- content of programme
- nature of delivery
- how people are going to be invited/referred to the group
- whether to include an induction week
- the size of the group

Style
Consider:

- Which educational style will be used
  - o experiential learning or didactic teaching
- What measures are required to ensure confidentiality
  - o safeguards will need to be in place

Knowledge and skills of group leader
Consider whether group leaders are:

- Competent to facilitate Behaviour Change Skills in a group setting
- Competent to manage group processes effectively (Group Facilitation Skills)
- Have up-to-date evidence-based knowledge on diet and activity

Time and resources
Consider whether:

- Sufficient time has been allocated for the planning, running and evaluation of the group programme, as well as administration time
- Suitable resources are available
- Adequate administration support is in place

Evaluation
Consider how best to evaluate the programme:

- What outcomes to measure: weight loss, clinical measurements, etc
- Patient Reported Outcome Measures (PROMS) – see Chapter 11
- Patient Reported Experience Measures (PREMS) – see Chapter 11
- Safety – are there any potential harmful effects for the individual? see Chapter 11
- Attendance rates
- Give consideration to long-term outcomes such as weight lost maintained at 1, 2 and 5 years

The above list is not exhaustive, but reflects the additional skill set needed to develop and deliver group-based programmes for weight management.

Commercial and self-help programmes

NICE suggests primary-care and local authorities recommend self-help, commercial and community weight-management programmes only if they adhere to best practice. This includes programmes which:

- Help people assess their weight and decide on a realistic healthy target weight loss (usually 5–10%)
- Aim for maximum weekly weight losses of 0.5–1.0 kg
- Focus on long-term lifestyle changes rather than short-term, quick-fix approaches.
- Are multicomponent, addressing diet and activity, and offering a variety of approaches
- Use a balanced, healthy-eating approach
- Recommend regular physical activity (particularly activities that can be part of daily life, such as brisk walking and gardening) and offer practical, safe advice about being more active
- Include some behaviour-change techniques, such as keeping a diary and advice on how to cope with 'lapses' and 'high-risk' situations
- Recommend and/or providing ongoing support

Group-based programmes are a potentially effective option for weight management when matched to the needs of the patient, but they require careful planning and need to be delivered by practitioners specifically trained in group-based skills. Group treatment does not replace the need for a comprehensive individual assessment, which is an essential stage in exploring treatment options and determining the most appropriate way forward. As group programmes are developed in the future, more attention needs to be given to ensuring protected time for their delivery and extended access [23].

Consider this

- Do you currently run groups?
- Are you fully equipped with the knowledge and skills required?
- Do you evaluate the effectiveness of the group?
- Do you refer to other weight-management groups?
- Are you familiar with the details of those groups?
- Do know how effective the programme is?

Drug treatment

The decision to start drug treatment, and the choice of drug, should be made after discussing with the patient the potential benefits and limitations, including the mode of action, adverse effects and monitoring requirements and their potential impact on the patient's motivation (see Chapter 3).

Surgery

Bariatric surgery is an option in severely obese patients, where lifestyle and medication have been tried but have proved ineffective. There are clear guidelines from NICE about who should be considered for bariatric surgery, although local criteria may differ from these depending on available resources (see Chapter 3).

Regardless of whether drug treatment or surgery is the chosen option, lifestyle treatment still remains central to maximizing outcomes achieved.

Conclusion

There are many different aspects to providing a comprehensive weight-management service. Decisions will be influenced by the needs of the local community, as well as local expertise and the resources available. Future planning needs to address any shortfalls in service to ensure that the needs of individuals within the local population are met.

Consider this

- Do you have responsibility for the provision of a weight-management service?
- Are the needs of your patient group being met?
- Are there any shortfalls in the provision of the service?
- How might the service be improved?

References

1. National Institute for Clinical Excellence. Obesity: Guidance on the Prevention, Identification, Assessment and Management of Overweight and Obesity in Adults and Children. NICE; 2006.
2. Stewart M, Brown J, Weston W, Mc Whinney I, McWilliams C, Freeman T, editors. Patient Centred Medicine Transforming the Clinical Method. Sage; 1995.
3. Rollnick S, Butler CC, Kinnersley P, Gregory J, Mash B. Motivational interviewing. BMJ 2010;340:c1900.
4. Cormier S, Nurius PS, Osborn CJ, editors. Interviewing and Change Strategies for Helpers. 6th edition. Belmont, CA: Brooks and Cole; 2009.
5. Scottish Intercollegiate Guidelines Network. Obesity in Scotland 2010. A National Guideline for Use in Scotland. Edinburgh: SIGN; 2010.
6. Miller WR, Rollnick S. Preparing people for change. In: Miller WR, Rollnick S, editors. Motivational Interviewing. Guilford Press; 2002.
7. Miller WR, Rollnick S. Ten things that motivational interviewing is not. Behav Cogn Psychother 2009 Mar;37[2]:129–40.
8. Rollnick S, Mason P, Butler C. Health Behaviour Change. A Guide for Practitioners. Churchill Livingstone; 1999.
9. Department of Health. Data Revisions Policy for the NHS Performance Monitoring Data. Local Data on Body Mass Index; 2010. Available from: http://www.dh.gov.uk/en/Publichealth/Obesity/DH_064011.

10. Department of Health. Healthy Weight, Healthy Lives: A Toolkit for Developing Local Strategies; 2008.

11. Department of Health. Department of Health Adult Care Pathway (Primary Care); 2006.

12. National Obesity Forum. Obesity Care Pathway. Available from: http://www.nationalobesityforum.org.uk/index.php/healthcare-professionals.html.

13. Public Health Action Support Team. Obesity Care Pathway Support Package; 2010. Available from: http://www.healthknowledge.org.uk/interactive-learning/obesity.

14. Royal College of Physicians. The Training of Health Professionals for the Prevention and Treatment of Overweight and Obesity; 2010

15. National Heart Lung and Blood Institute. Clinical Guidelines on the Identification, Evaluation and Treatment of Overweight and Obesity in Adults: The Evidence Report. National Institute of Health; 1998.

16. Latner JD, Stunkard AJ, Wilson GT, Jackson ML, Zelitch DS, Labouvie E. Effective long-term treatment of obesity: a continuing care model. Int J Obes Relat Metab Disord 2000 Jul;24[7]:893–8.

17. Bray GA. Obesity is a chronic, relapsing neurochemical disease. Int J Obes Relat Metab Disord 2004 Jan;28[1]:34–8.

18. Wing R. Behavioural approaches to the treatment of obesity In: Bray GA, Bouchard C, editors. Handbook of Obesity: Clinical Applications. New York: Marcel Dekker; 2004. pp. 147–67.

19. Cavill N, Hillsdon M, Antiss T. Brief Interventions for Weight Management. Oxford: National Obesity Observatory; 2011.

20. Laws R. Current approaches to obesity management in UK Primary Care: the Counterweight Programme. J Hum Nutr Diet 2004 Jun;17[3]:183–90.

21. Ebhohimhen VP, Avenell A. A systematic review of the effectiveness of group versus individual treatments for adult obesity. Obesity Facts 2009;2[1]:17–24.

22. Renjilian DA, Perri MG, Nezu AM, McKelvey WF, Shermer RL, Anton SD. Individual versus group therapy for obesity: effects of matching participants to their treatment preferences. J Consult Clin Psychol 2001 Aug;69[4]:717–21.

23. Allan K, Hoddinott P, Avenell A. A qualitative study comparing commercial and health service weight loss groups, classes and clubs. J Hum Nutr Diet 2011 Feb;24[1]:23–31.

6 Building a Picture: The Assessment

'Seek first to understand, then to be understood.'

St Francis of Assisi

Undertaking a comprehensive assessment

Weight management needs to be tailored to the individual [1,2]. This can only occur if a comprehensive assessment has been undertaken.

Traditionally, assessment has focused on clinical measurements such as height, weight, BMI and, more recently, waist measurement. While it is important to capture clinical data, it is equally important for the patient and practitioner to build a picture of the patient's past history and the current scenario. This includes exploring weight history, previous attempts to manage weight, motivation, barriers to change, current activity and eating patterns. The assessment also involves taking measurements of height, weight, waist (if BMI is under 35), blood pressure, lipid profile and blood glucose. Further tests may be included, depending on the medical picture.

'Going through everything with the nurse has really helped me understand much more about my weight.'

What are the components of the assessment?

This section aims to explore each component of the assessment:

1 The Beginning – getting started on the right footing
2 The Story So Far – developing an understanding of what has happened to date
3 Dealing with Expectations – of weight loss, its impact and the service
4 The Here and Now – ensuring that the current picture is complete and clear
5 The Ending – pulling it all together

Weight Management: A Practitioner's Guide, First Edition. Dympna Pearson and Clare Grace.
© 2012 Dympna Pearson and Clare Grace. Published 2012 by Blackwell Publishing Ltd.

The Beginning

Introductions

In a busy clinic it is easy to forget what the experience is like for the patient. Often overlooked are the vital elements which help build rapport at the beginning of the consultation:

- Meeting the patient in the waiting room, greeting them by name, and taking them through to the consultation room
- Inviting them to sit down and allowing them time to settle by engaging in some small talk
- Introducing yourself and checking the patient's details and preferred name
- Informing the patient of the time available for the consultation and checking if that is all right with them

Dialogue example

Practitioner: '*Welcome, my name is —. Can I check your details* [name, date of birth]? *What is your preferred name?*'
'*We are scheduled to finish at —. Is that ok for you?*'
'*I have had a letter from your doctor asking for you to be seen at this clinic. Would you mind filling me in on what led to him making that suggestion, from your point of view?*'
Patient: '*I went with headaches and he found I had high blood pressure and he said losing weight would help, so he suggested I come here.*'

Exploring importance (helps build motivation)

It should be established prior to starting any assessment that the patient is interested in losing weight and willing to commit to the programme. To build and strengthen motivation and facilitate change, the practitioner should encourage the patient to talk about their reasons for wanting to change – what makes weight change important to the individual?

Example of exploring importance

Practitioner: '*I wonder what your reaction was* [to the doctor suggesting that you lose weight].'
Patient: '*Well, I know it has crept up over the past few years, but I didn't realise it was affecting my health.*'
Practitioner: '*It sounds as if you are keen to do something about your weight?*'
Patient: '*Definitely, but it isn't easy!*'
Practitioner: '*As you say, losing weight is hard work and requires a lot of effort and commitment. It is helpful to be clear in your own mind why this is important for you. Thinking through your reasons for making this commitment can be really useful, especially when the going gets tough! It can help to remind yourself of why you are doing this. Can I ask you what makes it important for you?*'
Patient: '*Well, I know it is better for my health, but also, I want to feel better about myself, be fitter and able to wear nice clothes.*'
Practitioner: '*So, besides your health, you have a number of personal reasons for wanting to lose weight.*'
Patient: '*Yes, definitely!*'

The Story So Far

History of weight

It is important to gain a history of how the patient has reached their current weight, any major influences on weight and what has been happening recently. This conversation often highlights the patient's beliefs about their weight and what has influenced it.

> **Example of discussion about weight history**
>
> Practitioner: *'Perhaps we can start by you filling me in on what has happened with your weight in the past?'*
> Patient: *'Well, I started to put weight on when —.'*
> Practitioner: *'Your weight started to creep on when —. Can I ask you what has been happening recently?'*

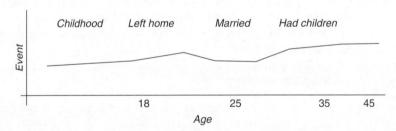

'I have put the weight on since I changed my job.'

'When the doctor came to see me in hospital, he told me to lose weight. He didn't know that I had already lost 2 stones!'

It is useful to encourage patients to reflect on their weight history in order to gain an understanding of what led to weight gain. Some people find it useful to capture their weight history on paper (Figure 6.1). This helps see when weight increased and whether it was related to a significant life event (see Tool 1).

Figure 6.1   Weight changes over time.

Previous attempts

> **Example of discussion about previous attempts**
>
> Practitioner: *'Can I ask if you have tried to lose weight before?'*
> Patient: *'I have tried everything – you name it, every diet under the sun, as well as all the slimming clubs.'*
> Practitioner: *'You have really tried and you sound very fed up that you haven't got the results you would like?'*

> Patient: '*I sometimes think I'm just one of those people who can't lose weight!*'
> Practitioner: '*Can I ask if any of what you tried worked?*'
> Patient: '*Well, yes, but only when I stayed on the diet. The minute I stopped, the weight came back on – it is so disheartening!*'

Many patients will have made numerous previous attempts to lose weight, but not all. It is important to capture this and acknowledge any previous efforts.

Weight cycling
Weight cycling is the repeated voluntary loss and subsequent regain of body weight in those who regularly follow weight-loss regimens. It is very common and is linked to increased health risks. Ideally, patients are trying to achieve sustainable lifestyle changes [2] and it can be helpful to capture the history of previous attempts and associated weight change.

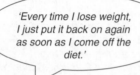

'*Every time I lose weight, I just put it back on again as soon as I come off the diet.*'

Understanding about weight

Patients often have strongly held beliefs about their weight: what has led to it increasing, what the causes are, and what works and doesn't work for them. It is important to discuss these as they arise. The genetic component often crops up during the assessment.

Discussing the genetic component
It is important to first listen to the patient's concerns, conveying empathy, and then explain the facts:

> **Example of discussion about genes**
>
> Patient: '*I think it is hopeless for me to try to lose weight – I just think it must be my genes. All my family are overweight and no matter what I do, I just can't lose weight!*'
> Practitioner: '*You sound fed up with trying to lose weight?*'
> Patient: '*Yes, well, I know lots of people who eat far more than me and they don't have a weight problem.*'
> Practitioner: '*It is very frustrating for you, looking at other people who don't seem to struggle like you do.*'
> Patient: '*Exactly!*'
> Practitioner: '*Would you like me to explain a bit about that?*'
> Patient: '*Yes.*'
> Practitioner: '*It seems there IS something in what you have observed. There has been a lot of research done in this area and it has been found that some people put weight on more easily and also find it more difficult to lose weight – they have the "fat-friendly genes"*'
> Patient: '*I knew it!*'
> Practitioner: '*There is some good news attached to this story.*'

Patient: *'Oh, yeah?'*
Practitioner: *'They have also found that even if you have the "fat-friendly genes", it is still possible to lose weight. It means you have to work hard at it and that is why we offer support, especially for someone like you, who finds it difficult.'*
Patient: *'You mean I'm not a hopeless case?'*
Practitioner: *'Provided you are happy to do the hard work at home, I will give you all the support I can.'*
Patient: *'Great, when can I start?!'*

Dealing with Expectations

There are many expectations linked to weight loss which need to be explored.

Weight loss

Example of discussion about weight loss expectations

Practitioner: *'Have you thought about how much weight you would like to lose?'*
Patient: *'I need to lose at least 3 stones!'*
Practitioner: *'3 stones would be an amazing weight loss and that might be possible over a long period of time. However, I find it helpful to look at what is realistic in the short-term. Would you like me to tell you what I have in mind?'*
Patient: *'Sure.'*
Practitioner: *'For your current weight [11½ stones] the experts recommend aiming for 1½ stones over the first 3–6 months at the rate of 1–2 pounds per week and then taking stock – in other words, approaching weight loss in a stepwise fashion. How does that sound to you?'*
Patient: *'OK, but I need to lose more than 1½ stones!'*
Practitioner: *'Individuals vary on what they achieve and it may be possible over a period of time. How about we review progress as you go along, initially aiming for 1½ stones over the next 3 months and then we can take stock?'*

Many patients have unrealistic expectations about the amount of weight they are likely to lose during a weight-management intervention. Although amounts and rates of weight loss vary from one person to another, research shows average weight losses with conservative lifestyle approaches tend not to exceed 10% of initial weight. This is one of the most difficult aspects of weight management. Understandably, practitioners do not like to dampen enthusiasm, especially in the early stages, and patients are reluctant to accept they may not reach their 'ideal weight'. Sensitive and skilful handling of this topic is essential to reaching a stage where the patient accepts an 'altered' target weight. Acceptance of a body weight that is not necessarily 'ideal' has been suggested as an important factor in preventing weight regain [3]. Initial weight-management targets should aim for 5–10% of starting weight over 3–6 months. Thereafter, a joint decision can be made about whether to have a period of weight maintenance and consolidation or whether further weight loss is advisable. Six months seems to be a 'window of opportunity' during which maximum weight loss can be achieved, so effort needs to focus on achieving maximum results during this period.

Benefits of losing weight

How does the patient see weight loss affecting them? Some people believe it will change everything in their life and it is important to realistically address what weight loss can and cannot achieve. This may need to be addressed over time and people with serious underlying difficulties (such as relationship problems) may need to be referred for appropriate help.

Expectations of the service

If it has not already been covered, the details of the service on offer should be explained:

- Frequency and duration of appointments
- The content of the sessions
- The approach used, e.g. self-monitoring and practising new skills in between appointments

Example of discussion about the service

Summarise the conversation so far:

Practitioner: 'So far we have looked at what led to you coming today and what has been happening with your weight and the things you have tried to date. You have really tried hard and nothing seems to have worked – is that right?'
Patient: 'Yes. To be honest, I'm fed up with the whole thing.'
Practitioner: 'You sound really frustrated that all the effort you have made has not given you the results you would like?'
Patient: 'Yes, that's it!'
Practitioner: 'Would it be helpful if I explained about this service and what it offers?'
Patient: 'Yes, please.'
Practitioner: 'Today's appointment is an opportunity to capture what has been happening so far for you in relation to your weight. We can discuss what you are hoping to gain from attending as well as making sure we have all the relevant medical details. Once we have a clear picture, we can then think about the best options for you. How does all that sound?'
Patient: 'Fine'.
Practioner: 'Is there anything you would like to ask?'

Patients are often unclear about services on offer and it helps to clarify this at the beginning. This also provides the opportunity for the patient to consider what is available and decide whether this meets their needs and if they are willing and able to commit to the programme (*exploring motivation*).

What the practitioner can offer

It is important to be clear about the support which can be provided by the practitioner.

> **Example of discussion about support practitioner can offer**
>
> Practitioner: *'Would you like me to outline what support I can offer?'*
> Patient: *'Yes, please.'*
> Practitioner: *'After today, if you decide that this is something you really want to go ahead with, we can draw up a plan for regular appointments. I would like to offer you X appointments over the next 3 months. [This will vary depending on resource]. We can then review progress and decide what suits best at that point. Are you happy with that?'*

Patient commitment

It is also important to be clear about the level of commitment required from the patient and what this might mean in practice. This links with patient **consent** and the development of a common agenda.

> **Example of establishing patient commitment**
>
> Practitioner: *'The hard work is done by you in between appointment, but I am here to support you at each visit. We can work through any difficulties you may be experiencing. It does require a commitment from you to attend on a regular basis. I can try to fit the appointments in with your schedule* [or appointments are at — time]. *How does that sound?'*
> Patient: *'Do you think I need to come that often?'*
> Practitioner: *'Yes, research shows that people who attend regular appointments do best. At each appointment, we will review progress and address any difficulties that you may be experiencing, and at each session we will cover a specific topic* [from this list – show 'Menu of Options' chart, Tools 8–10] *to ensure that you are well equipped with the necessary knowledge and skills to not only help you lose weight but keep it off long-term. Are you happy to proceed?'* **[Seeking consent]**
> Patient: *'Yes! It looks like there is a lot to cover. What happens now?'*
> Practitioner: *'We can continue to develop a complete picture.'*

The Here and Now

At this stage, try to aim for an overview of current eating and activity habits. Do not be tempted to focus prematurely on detail, which can be gathered through self-monitoring as the intervention proceeds.

Establishing current eating habits

The assessment needs to consider how food fits into the person's life. At this early stage it is helpful to map out an overall picture of meal patterns, types of foods eaten and what influences food choice, rather than focusing on the detail of exactly what is eaten. Ask the patient to describe how food fits into a Typical Day (Table 6.1) and follow the description in a nonjudgmental way using reflective listening skills. Many health professionals complain that patients do not tell the truth about what they eat. It is true that people generally underestimate what they eat and there are many reasons for this, including poor awareness of dietary intake and reluctance to be open with someone else about what they are eating, often for fear of being judged. An overall view of how food fits into the person's life is usually sufficient to guide the initial steps needed for effective weight management. Food diaries can then be used to gain a more accurate record of food intake over time (see Chapter 7, page 113–117).

Table 6.1   Example of a typical day

Time	Food	Activity
7am	Cup of Tea	
8am	Breakfast: Bowl of cereal or toast	Dashing round getting kids ready for school Drop kids off at school & drive to work
9am	Coffee	Office – desk
10.30am	Coffee & biscuits	Office meeting
12.30pm	**Lunch:** Sandwich – different fillings Packet of Crisps, sometimes chocolate Cola	Working through lunch
2pm	Cup of tea & cake (if someone's birthday) or biscuit	Office – desk
3pm		Leave work to collect kids
4pm	Cup of tea & snack with kids e.g. biscuit or chocolate bar	After-school activities – car & waiting around
5.30pm		Preparing tea
6–6.30pm	**Evening Meal:** Pasta dish, bolognaise, chicken, pizza Chips or garlic bread Roast dinner on Sunday	Sit at kitchen table
8pm		Housework
9pm	Nibbles: crisps & maybe a glass of wine	Watch TV
10pm		Bedtime

Example of discussion about Typical Day

Practitioner: '*This seems like a good time to get a picture of how food fits in for you. Would you mind taking me through a typical day, describing what you have to eat and drink from when you get up in the morning, going right through the day?*'
Patient: '*Weekends are very different to weekdays.*'
Practitioner: '*Shall we focus on weekdays to begin with?*'
Patient: '*Well, mornings are really busy…*'

Try to follow the patient's description of their day in a nonjudgmental way, using reflective listening skills. Ideally, guide the conversation to obtain not only an overall view of how food fits in, but importantly the factors which influence the patient's food choices (see Table 6.1 and Tool 2).

NB Avoid asking lots of questions which risk turning the conversation into an interrogation!

It is important not to focus prematurely on details of types and quantities of foods. The task is to get an overall view and to help the patient become more aware of current food and drink intake and develop a common understanding. This continues to build rapport and the helping relationship.

Tip: It can be helpful to write down the patient's description (making sure that they can see what you write). It helps both the patient and practitioner to see as well as hear a clear picture. Also, it acts as a useful record when considering changes later.

Remember to thank the patient for going through this exercise, which can often be difficult for them. Also, it is worth asking if they would like to comment.

Example of asking for reflection on Typical Day

Practitioner: '*Thank you for going through that with me, it sounds as if you have a busy schedule! I wonder what your thoughts are having just gone through that* [sharing the written record].'
Patient: '*I can see I have too many snacks!*'
Practitioner: '*You think perhaps it is worth cutting down on snacks – that sounds like a good place to start! We can look at that in detail later when we come to developing your individual plan.*'

Binge eating

Compared to people without binge eating disorder (BED), those diagnosed with the condition are heavier, more likely to be overweight as a child, demonstrate weight cycling and have higher levels of psychological co-morbidity, including anxiety, depression and personality disorders [3]. Practitioners should be aware of the possibility of BED in patients who have difficulty losing weight and maintaining weight loss [2].

Questions exploring whether binge eating is a possibility need to be asked in a very sensitive manner as patients with this disorder may experience high levels of shame, embarrassment and guilt. It may not always be disclosed at the initial assessment, but later when a trusting relationship has been established.

It is important to try and establish whether what the patient is describing as binge eating falls within the diagnostic criteria. The screening for BED questionnaire (Appendix 7) can help indicate wheter a referral to an eating disorder service is indicated. For less severe cases, the use a self-help manual may be an effective strategy (Resource 15).

Establishing current level of activity

Physical activity is an essential component of any weight-management programme and is particularly important for weight maintenance. The majority of the population (both slim and overweight) is inactive and new physical activities adopted need to be sustainable. The starting point is to capture current levels of activity and inactivity. This can be done in a variety of ways. Initially, ask the patient about their level of activity:

Example of discussion about activity

Practitioner: *'Would you describe yourself as an active person?'*
Patient: *'Yes, I'm on the go all the time!'*
Practitioner: *'Would you mind telling me about the kind of things that keep you busy?'*
Patient: *'Work, running round after the kids – I'm a glorified taxi-driver!'*
Practitioner: *'They keep you busy! Any sports activities that you enjoy?'*
Patient: *'I used to play netball, but I just don't have time. I joined the gym after Christmas but I stopped going...'*
Practitioner: *'It sounds as if you really find it hard to fit in anything extra?'*
Patient: *'Exactly!'*

Safety

The General Practice Physical Activity Questionnaire (GPPAQ) (Appendix 8) [5] and the Physical Activity Readiness Questionnaire (PAR-Q) (Appendix 9) [2] are quick, validated tools for determining whether individuals require additional investigations prior to embarking on a programme of increased physical activity.

Exploring possible difficulties (helps builds confidence and motivation)

A patient's belief in their ability to lose weight can be a major stumbling block to successful weight management. There are various reasons for this, including: past experiences, lack of cooking, shopping and menu-planning skills, low income, tensions across family and social situations, perceived lack of willpower and so on.

The task of the practitioner is to help build confidence and the patient's belief in their ability to succeed.

Example of establishing confidence in ability to be more active

Practitioner: *'Is making changes to your eating and activity something you feel able to take on at the moment?'*
Patient: *'I want to but it is difficult... I mean, I'm so busy, I don't have time for exercise.'*

It is important, as part of a thorough assessment, to establish current and/or past difficulties experienced by the patient in managing their weight. These actual and perceived difficulties need to be highlighted and explored.

Example of discussing obstacles to activity

Practitioner: *'Besides finding time for activity, is there anything that would make it difficult for you to lose weight?'*
Patient: *'Fitting it in at home with everyone else's likes and dislikes – it's a nightmare!'*
Practitioner: *'Would it be helpful if we look at some ideas on how you might get round that once we have the complete picture?'*
Patient: *'Yes, I need some ideas!'*
Practitioner: *'Is there anything else?'*
Patient: *'Not that I can think of...'*

Establishing the clinical picture – medical/clinical measurements

Key components of the clinical assessment

- Weight
- Height
- BMI
- Waist (BMI under 35)
- Blood Pressure
- Bloods: blood glucose, lipids, U & Es, LFTs, thyroid function
- Medical history
- Medications
- Risk factors.

Medical examination
This should include measurement of height (Appendix 2) and weight (Appendix 3) and calculation of BMI (Appendix 4). Waist measurement (Appendix 5) can be used in addition to BMI, as a predictor of risk of metabolic and vascular complications for those with a BMI of 35 or below [1]. Waist measurement does not add any additional information for those with a BMI above 35 [2]. Check for conditions linked with obesity, such as sleep apnoea, menstrual disturbances, depression and joint or back pain. Video resources for height, weight and waist measurements are Resources 10–12.

Investigations
Blood-pressure measurements and blood tests should be taken to identify associated health risks or co-morbidities, such as impaired glucose tolerance, type 2 diabetes and lipid, thyroid, liver and/or renal abnormalities.

Medical history
It is important to ascertain any other medical problems that should not be neglected during a weight-management intervention.

Medications
A number of medications are associated with weight gain [2] (Appendix 6) and it is important to document and discuss the implications of these with the patient.

Risk factors

The clinical assessment should highlight the presence of associated co-morbidities such as established coronary heart disease, atherosclerosis, impaired glucose tolerance, type 2 diabetes, gynaecological problems, osteoarthritis, gallstones, stress incontinence and cardiovascular risk factors such as smoking, hypertension, hyperlipidaemia and a family history of CHD. Those patients who have been identified as having **metabolic syndrome** should be highlighted for intensive treatment for the prevention of CHD and stroke.

Metabolic syndrome: This is a group of risk factors, including central obesity, dyslipidaemia and hypertension, that are strongly associated with type 2 diabetes and significantly greater risks of cardiovascular disease. Coronary heart disease and stroke are approximately doubled and the risk of death from coronary heart disease is four-fold [4].

Cut-off points for Metabolic Syndrome

The presence of **three or more** of the following four symptoms in the same individual indicates the metabolic syndrome [2]:

1　**Blood pressure ≥ 130/85 mm Hg or on BP medication**
2　**Type 2 diabetes or impaired glucose tolerance or FBG ≥ 5.6 mmol/l**
3　**Being overweight or obese/excess body fat, particularly around the waist**
　　○　a waistline of 102 cm or more for men (90 cm for Asian men) and 88 cm or more for women (80 cm in Asian women)
4　**Impaired lipid profile**
　　○　triglycerides ≥ 1.7 mmol/l or HDL cholesterol < 1.03 in men or < 1.29 in women

The WHO defines metabolic syndrome as **three** or **more** of the four symptoms listed above and [5]

5　**Microalbuminuria ≤ 20 g/min or albumin: creatinine ratio ≤ 30 mg**

Clinical tests may be completed prior to the assessment consultation or by another member of the team. It is important that these are undertaken in a sensitive person-centred manner.

The Ending

Assessment provides the opportunity to gather crucial information on the patient's weight, health and lifestyle. It is also an opportunity to establish and build on the helping relationship. Conducting an assessment in a conversational way, using good interpersonal skills to accurately capture and reflect what the patient is saying, is likely to elicit improved understanding of their story, minimise the resistance to change and enhance the therapeutic relationship. By guiding the conversation in a way that makes the patient feel comfortable, the practitioner facilitates a consultation which should end with a shared view and a common agenda.

NB Some services use a template to complete the assessment. These can provide helpful prompts for practitioners but may feel like an interrogation for the patients unless they are used in a patient-centred way.

A thorough assessment can take 45–60 minutes.

If time is limited, it can be completed over a number of consultations.

Agreeing a way forward

When the assessment has been completed and the patient is happy to proceed with the intervention, it is time to move on to **explore options and find solutions** for changing activity and eating habits.

Consider this

You have just completed an assessment with an overweight patient.
- Have you got a complete picture?
- Has the patient got a complete picture?
- Is there a common understanding?
- Have you got a common agenda?
- Have you got a plan for the way forward?
- Has a good rapport been built?

References

1. National Institute for Clinical Excellence. Obesity: Guidance on the Prevention, Identification, Assessment and Management of Overweight and Obesity in Adults and Children. NICE; 2006.
2. Scottish Intercollegiate Guidelines Network. Management of Obesity: A National Clinical Guideline. SIGN; 2010.
3. Bruce B, Wilfley D. Binge eating among the overweight population: a serious and prevalent problem. J Am Diet Assoc 1996 Jan;96[1]:58–61.
4. Sattar N, Gaw A, Scherbakova O, Ford I, O'Reilly DS, Haffner SM, et al. Metabolic syndrome with and without C-reactive protein as a predictor of coronary heart disease and diabetes in the West of Scotland Coronary Prevention Study. Circulation 2003 Jul 29;108[4]:414–19.
5. World Health Organization. Definition, Diagnosis and Classification of Diabetes Mellitus and its Complications; 1999.

7 Finding Solutions: Supporting Patients to Establish a Solid Foundation

'We can't solve problems by using the same kind of thinking we used when we created them.'

Albert Einstein

Introduction

This chapter focuses on the initial stages of weight management. The first few consultations should support patients to establish a solid foundation of knowledge and skills essential to lifelong weight management. Once this has been achieved, patients can build on developing additional expertise as outlined in Chapter 8. Patients begin weight-management attempts with varying degrees of knowledge and skills. Working in this structured way ensures everyone has the same solid foundation of information and skills, although clearly there will be patients who can progress more quickly.

Integrating a behavioural approach

Problem-solving is central to a behavioural approach and developing problem-solving skills for weight management is essential for individuals who struggle with their weight. A very effective way of helping people to develop this skill is to model the process during consultations, working in a collaborative way. This section outlines how a problem-solving approach can be integrated.

Problem-solving process

Step 1: Identify the problem
Step 2: Explore options
Step 3: Choose preferred options
Step 4: Develop a plan
Step 5: Implement the plan
Step 6: Review the plan

Weight Management: A Practitioner's Guide, First Edition. Dympna Pearson and Clare Grace.
© 2012 Dympna Pearson and Clare Grace. Published 2012 by Blackwell Publishing Ltd.

Step 1: Identify the Problem

This step is undertaken through the process of completing an **assessment** in a collaborative manner as detailed in Chapter 6. It helps to gain a complete picture and identify problem areas, which can then be explored before moving on to finding solutions. There will be ongoing assessment throughout the intervention. **Self-monitoring** is an invaluable tool for raising awareness and highlighting difficulties.

Step 2: Explore Options

Explore as many options as possible and encourage patients to be creative.

Example of exploring dietary options

Practitioner: '*Shall we look at the recommendations for weight loss from the food side of things?*'
Patient: '*I guess it is a case of 'eat less …'*'
Practitioner: '*Yes and there are a number of other important points to consider as well.*'
Patient: '*Such as …?*'
Practitioner: '*Well as the goal is not only to lose weight but to keep it off, there are a couple of other points that are helpful to consider.*'
Patient: '*Oh yes?*'
Practitioner: '*Regular meals are seen as being a vital foundation for managing your weight. It is also important to make sure that your diet is nutritionally adequate especially as weight management is lifelong – another "foundation stone" that needs to be in place!*'
Patient: '*Mm I see.*'
Practitioner: '*Could we look at your food intake during a typical day [see Chapter 6] and see how it compares with those recommendations and then we can focus on reducing the calories?*'
Patient: '*OK.*'

Exploring physical activity options

Practitioner: '*Would it be useful if we now look at the recommendations for activity?*'
Patient: '*OK.*'
Practitioner: '*Well, firstly, the experts are now distinguishing between activity and inactivity. They recommend that we try to reduce the amount of time spent sitting, such as watching TV, driving, sitting at desks and so on.*'
Patient: '*I do enough of that!*'
Practitioner: '*You might find it useful to fill in this chart to establish how much of your time is spent sitting [Tool 3]. You can then look at how you might break that up. It is recommended that we do not sit for longer than half an hour, if possible. You might be interested to see how you compare with that?*'
Patient: '*OK, what about exercise? I hope you are not going to tell me to go to the gym!*'
Practitioner: '*Again, it would be useful to see where your starting point is and you can build from that.*'
Patient: '*Makes sense!*'
Practitioner: '*One easy way of doing that would be to use a pedometer to count your daily steps.*' [Explain about using a pedometer or suggest recording activity in minutes.]

Step 3: Choose Preferred Option/s

Encourage patients to come up with their own suggestions, once they have information on what works best for weight loss. Some patients will happily volunteer suggestions, others may not. If not, the practitioner needs to make suggestions to guide the patient towards dietary changes that will achieve the desired weight loss.

NB Always ask permission before making suggestions. Otherwise, you are likely to meet the 'Yes, but ...' response.

A) Example of choosing preferred dietary option/s

Practitioner: *'Any comments from looking at your typical day?'*
Patient: *'I can see that my meals are all over the place.'*
Practitioner: *'Yes, it makes sense to put the foundations in place.*
Patient: *'I don't think my diet looks that healthy, either!'.'*
Practitioner: *'That is something you can aim to improve over time as well.'*
Patient: *'But will I lose weight?'*
Practitioner: *'For that to happen, it is important to ensure that the calories you are taking in are less that those you are using up, with your day-to-day activities. Anything in particular that you think you should change to cut down on your calorie intake?'*
Patient: *'I can see all the snacks need to go and some (not all!) of the booze.'*
Practitioner: *'You have mentioned quite a few things there; maybe we can develop a plan so that you are really clear about what you are going to do?'*
Patient: *'Good idea!'*

B) Example of choosing preferred activity/inactivity option/s

Practitioner: *'Are you happy to make a note of the time spent sitting, driving, watching TV and so on? Or you could fill in this chart* [Tool 3].'
Patient: *'I'll fill in the chart – I like visual images.'*
Practitioner: *'Great! Now, to get an idea of your level of activity, which would you prefer – to use a pedometer or to keep a record of the number of minutes spent on different activities?'*
Patient: *'I think I'd like to try a pedometer.'*

Step 4: Develop a Plan

Planning ahead is necessary for successful change. Practitioners often say they use a goal-setting approach, when in reality they help patients set targets, such as 'eat breakfast' or 'cut down on fats'. Patients find it difficult to translate consultation-room discussions into action. The theory of setting **SMART goals** is well understood by health care professionals, but putting it into practice is another matter. Helping patients develop a detailed personal action plan is more likely to succeed – the **what, how** and **when** of change. Encourage patients to think through the details of how they are going to implement their plan in everyday life.

Plan, plan, plan – the secret of success!

Example of discussing a detailed diet plan

Practitioner: *'Shall we look at the first target you have set yourself?'*
Patient: *'Yes. That's trying to eat more regular meals and not to skip breakfast.'*
Practitioner: *'It is a really good idea to think this through in some detail and capture it on paper – is that OK?'*
Patient: *'Sure.'*

Talk through with patients the detail of their plan. Cover **what** is going to change and **how** this will be achieved. Discuss **what** might get in the way of changes and **how** to overcome any difficulties. Once this exercise has been completed, encourage patients to use the same approach for all changes they intend to make. The practitioner is helping patients develop their goal-setting skills by going through this process. It should be reviewed and repeated, if necessary on follow-up appointments (see Tool 4).

The more detailed the plan, the better!

Example of a *food* Change Plan

What change am I going to make?   *'Have breakfast each day.'*
How am I going to make sure it happens?

1 *'Get up when the alarm goes off!'*
2 *'Leave cereal, dish and spoon on the table the night before.'*
3 *'Ask my wife to buy suitable cereal.'*
4 *'Increase the milk order from the milkman and change to semi-skimmed.'*

What might get in the way?   *'Turning over when the alarm goes off!'*
How will I get round that?   *'Move the alarm clock to where I cannot reach!'*
When will I start?   *'Monday morning.'*

Encourage patients to imagine making the changes. e.g. *'Can you imagine yourself doing that each day?'*

Example of an *activity* Change Plan

What change am I going to make?   *'Go for a 30-minute walk each day.'*
How am I going to make sure it   *'Take a 15 minute walk at lunchtime and*
happens?   *15 minutes in the evening.'*

1 *'Let people at work know that this is my new routine.'*
2 *'Bring a comfortable pair of shoes to the office and leave under my desk.'*
3 *'Ask my wife to encourage me to go for a walk after the evening meal.'*
4 *'If I miss it, make up the time at weekends.'*

What might get in the way?   *'Being busy at work and tired in the evenings!'*
How will I get round that?   *'Ask people around me to provide encouragement.'*
When will I start?   *'Tomorrow.'*

Encourage patients to imagine making the changes. e.g. *'Can you imagine yourself doing that each day?'*

> *'Learning the importance of developing a detailed plan has really helped me.'*

Enlisting support

Enlisting **support** and finding ways of using **rewards** to reinforce new habits (see Chapter 8) should be included as part of developing a plan. This needs to be an ongoing process and should be included in review appointments.

It can be helpful to compare the development of a Change Plan with an activity the person is familiar with in everyday life, such as gardening or decorating. In order to successfully complete many everyday activities, a detailed plan is needed. Sometimes relating weight-management plans to those developed in other aspects of a patient's life can be helpful.

Step 5: Implement the Plan

Given it is the patient who implements the plan outside the consultation room, it is essential they have a clear idea of what to do and how to do it. Helping them to visualise carrying out the plan at home by talking through the detail and considering possible difficulties and how they might deal with setbacks is likely to be helpful in achieving success. This should be an ongoing process, along with self-monitoring, an important tool in identifying problems as they occur. The subsequent generation of solutions may come from the patient, or from their working collaboratively with the practitioner at review appointments.

Example of a discussion about implementing a diet plan

Practitioner: *'Now you have a detailed plan for both eating and activity, can you envisage it all falling into place at home?'*
Patient: *'I think so.'*
Practitioner: *'I guess the best way to find out is to give it a go. Anything that we haven't thought about can be discussed at your next appointment. It is rare for someone to lose weight without having some slip-ups along the way. That is why attending on a regular basis is so important – we can address any difficulties as we go along. Think of your plan as "work in progress" that will need tweaking as we go.'*
Patient: *'That makes sense.'*
Practitioner: *'Can we think about how you are going to monitor progress?'*
Patient: *'How do you mean?'*
Practitioner: *'It seems that people who record progress do better than those who don't. Is it something you would be happy to do?'*
Patient: *'I guess so, if it helps'.*
Practitioner: *'Do you have any thoughts on how you might like to do this?'* [See more on self-monitoring later in this chapter.]

Step 6: Review the Plan

This final step reviews progress, sets new goals and adapts the plan. The practitioner supports the patient during this process, continues to provide information and helps the patient develop the necessary skills to manage their weight long-term.

Follow-up appointments are an opportunity to review progress and set new goals, and for the practitioner to guide the patient to expand beyond the initial knowledge and skills vital for long-term success. Effective appointments are structured and patients benefit from being fully informed of programme details, such as how many visits are involved, how frequently and over what time period, and the duration of each consultation. It is recommended that patients are seen initially over a 6-month period (weekly or biweekly), with each appointment requiring a minimum of 10–15 minutes. Appointments can be spread over a longer period if good progress is being made, although this will depend to some degree on local resources. It is vital that patients are clear on what to expect and that agreement is reached on how review appointments are to be organised.

Consider this

You have just helped a patient develop a plan for weight loss.
Is **the plan**:

S – Specific (What exactly are they going to change?)
M – Measurable (Can the change be measured?)
A – Achievable (Is this plan going to be possible for this patient?)
R – Realistic (Are the planned changes realistic and likely to fit in?)
T – Time-specific (When is it going to start?)

If the plan focuses on the **what**, **how** and **when** of change, it should be SMART.

Review appointments need to be **structured**:

- Review progress with changes to eating and activity (using a diary). Discuss what has gone well/not so well
  - Affirm success and offer encouragement
  - Discuss any difficulties using reflective listening skills
- Review progress with weight
  - Affirm success and encourage
  - Discuss any difficulties using reflective listening skills
- Explore options and set new goals, modifying the change plan
- Discuss support
- Discuss ways of reinforcing new habits (rewards or encouragers)
- Discuss a topic from the 'Menu of Options' and/or some strategies or skills required for weight management (see Chapter 8)

Review appointments: checklist for agreement with the patient

☐ Duration of weight-loss phase of treatment.
☐ Frequency of visits.
☐ Time allocated for each visit.
☐ Appointment times for first month.
☐ Need for continuous care and support during the weight-maintenance phase.
☐ Review progress at 3 and 6 months.

Review progress at 3 and 6 months

At 3 months:

- If no progress, consider medication or referral to specialist unit, depending on BMI
- Consider: 'Is the treatment working?' and if not, discuss appropriate action with the patient

At 6 months:

- Some patients may wish to continue with weight loss and need regular visits for support
- Some may wish to maintain the weight they have lost and still require ongoing support for weight maintenance
- Discuss whether the programme is suitable for the patient and is achieving agreed targets

If at any stage the patient exits the programme, ensure medical problems receive continuing care and that the patient continues to feel supported regardless of their weight

The building blocks needed for a solid foundation

A solid foundation for successfully managing weight requires a set of knowledge and skills built up over time.

The rest of this chapter focuses on providing information in a helpful way, key diet and physical activity recommendations, their practical application, and key skills required for implementation. Topics covered include:

- Understanding energy balance.
- Key dietary recommendations:
  o practical application of dietary messages.
- Recommendations for physical activity:
  o practical application of physical-activity messages.
- Developing essential skills: laying the foundations:
  o problem-solving skills
  o self-monitoring – keeping a diary
  o goal setting – developing a change plan.

'Bear in mind that any changes to eating and activity habits take time and need to be approached in a stepwise manner.'

Providing information in a helpful way – an essential practitioner skill

The ability of individuals to make informed choices about changes to eating and activity habits is essential to ensuring those changes are meaningful. The practitioner has a vital role in providing information on dietary and physical-activity recommendations that will facilitate sustained weight loss.

Providing information in a way that is appropriate requires a level of practitioner skill that is often underestimated. Finding the right words and phrases for different individuals in different situations requires practice and expertise.

Route map for providing information

- **Check** what the person already knows
- **Ask** if they would like some information
- **Provide** information in 'bite-sized' pieces as a two-way exchange (checking how the information is being received as you go along, allowing for comments and questions and observing nonverbal cues)
- **Check** what it means to the individual

'People are often confused by conflicting dietary messages – health care professionals need to ensure their messages are consistent with current evidence.'

Example of providing information

Practitioner: 'Are you clear about what is currently recommended for successful weight management?' **[Check]**
Patient: 'Isn't it just about eating less and exercising more?
Practitioner: 'That's it in a nutshell. Would you like me to go through what has been shown to work well?' **[Ask]**
Patient: 'Sure.'
Practitioner: 'It has been found that in order to lose weight and keep it off, it is necessary to make changes to eating and activity that can be maintained and that fit for each individual. That is what this programme offers: working with you as an individual to find what works best for you.' **[Provide]** 'How does that sound?' **[Check]**
Patient: 'Yes, it definitely has to fit in. Otherwise I won't be able to keep to it.'

Understanding energy balance

Calories in vs calories out

Weight loss is achieved through consuming fewer calories than are expended. A deficit of 500–600 kcals per day will result in weight loss of approximately 0.5 kg (1 lb) per week.

Thermodynamics of weight loss

3500 calories = 0.5 kg body fat
7000 calories = 1 kg body fat

Energy requirements:

Average man	2500 calories/day
Average woman	2000 calories/day

To lose weight:

Men	**Women**
2500 calories/day	2000 calories/day
–500 calories/day	– 500 calories/day ×7 = 3500 calories (= 0.5 kg body fat)
2000 calories/day	1500 calories/day

A calorie deficit can be achieved by a combination of decreased food intake and increased activity.

NB Calorie intake should not be reduced below 1200 per day to ensure nutritional adequacy of the diet, unless supervised by experienced medical and dietetic practitioners.

'The thing that helped me most was when I understood the "calories-in/calories-out" equation. After that, I realised the importance of tracking my daily calorie intake.'

Recommended rates of weight loss

For most people, weight loss of 2–3 kg (4–7 lb) per month is realistic. That is, '½ stone a month'.

How many calories?

1   Most men will lose at the recommended rate on 1800 calories/day.
2   Most women will lose at the recommended rate on 1500 calories/day.

People with higher BMIs lose weight on higher calorie intakes because their energy requirements are higher (see Appendices 10 or 11 to estimate individual energy requirements). Consider referral to specialist weight-management service (see local pathways).

Key dietary recommendations

The most effective dietary treatment for the management of weight is a hotly debated issue and subject to ongoing research. As new studies are published, they are sometimes misreported in the press, leading to confusion about which strategies are most effective. The dietary recommendations below outline where there is major consensus on the dietary approaches to weight management.

Recommendations for weight management based on current evidence

- Use a structured and coordinated approach [1]
- The main requirement of a dietary weight-management approach is to ensure total energy intake is less than energy expenditure [2,3]
- Dietary interventions for weight loss should be calculated to produce a 600 kcal/day energy deficit [2,3]
- Programmes should be tailored to the dietary preferences of the individual patient [2,3]
- When discussing dietary change with patients, health care professionals should emphasise achievable and sustainable healthy eating [2,3]

Initial steps towards achieving dietary recommendations

Encourage self-monitoring (keeping a daily record of food and drink intake) and explore the following:

Current eating patterns
Explore the frequency of meals and snacks.
Encourage regular meals.

A nutritionally adequate diet
Base food intake on the 'eatwell plate'.

Start by focusing on the **Frequency**, **Amount** and **Type** (**FAT**) of foods eaten. This will often automatically achieve a calorie deficit, as well as nutritional adequacy of the diet:

Frequency
Aim for food **proportions** to be similar to those on the 'eatwell plate' [2].

Amount
Develop awareness of suitable portion/serving sizes.

Type
Consider lower-calorie alternatives to foods eaten, e.g. semi-skimmed milk instead of full cream milk.

Learn how to read labels
Learn to read the **calorie** content on food labels in order to enable informed choices.

Record calorie intake
Learn what calories different foods provide in order to enable informed choices.

Compare calorie intake with weight loss achieved
Is the desired weight loss being achieved?

Encourage healthy eating as a way of life – essential for maintenance of weight lost and overall health benefits

How to commence self-monitoring to understand current eating patterns

Note on self-monitoring: Diary 1 (below) shows a patient who has recorded food intake from memory at the end of the day. Diary 2 (below) shows a patient who recorded as they went along through the day. Diary 2 is much more accurate and provides the patient with greater insight into current eating habits. **Research shows that the majority of people under-record (and therefore underestimate their food intake)** [4]. The task of the practitioner is to support patients practising the skill of more-accurate recording of their food intake. Once a clear picture has been established, the patient can move forward to establish a regular meal pattern in a stepwise manner. Remember, it can take time to change established eating habits.

Diary 1: patient recording meals and snacks

Breakfast	Tea & toast
Mid-morning	Coffee & biscuits
Lunch	Sandwich
Mid-afternoon	Tea & cake
Evening meal	Meat, vegetables & potato
During the evening	Crisps, chocolate and wine

*Estimated calorie content: 1200 kcals

Diary 2: patient recording frequency

8 am	Tea
8.15 am	Toast & butter & jam
9 am	Coffee & chocolates from office tin
10 am	Coffee & biscuits
12.30 pm	Egg mayo sandwich & smoothie
1.30 pm	½ chocolate bar
3 pm	Tea & lemon cake
5 pm	Apple
6 pm	Chunk of cheese
7 pm	Meat, veg & potato
7.30 pm	Yogurt
8 pm	Crisps and wine
9.30 pm	Bar of chocolate
10 pm	Tea

*Estimated calorie content: 2000 kcals

'I am amazed how much more accureate my food diary is when I write things down as I go along.'

How to encourage regular eating

1 Encourage regular meals, including breakfast, lunch, evening meal and snacks (if appropriate)
2 Avoid long gaps between meals or fasting. A sensible guide is 4–5 hours between meals and 2–3 hours between snacks
3 Avoid grazing or frequent snacking
4 Avoid binge eating. Long fasts usually lead to overconsumption

How to ensure a nutritionally adequate diet

Eating healthily is important due to its influence on reducing the risk of chronic diseases as well as in order to promote health and well being. A healthy diet reduces the risk of coronary heart disease, stroke, type 2 diabetes, osteoporosis and some cancers. Eating healthily provides the energy and nutrients for the various bodily systems to function optimally. Practitioners working in weight management need to support patients to establish and sustain healthy eating habits and ensure the diet is adequate in terms of macronutrients (carbohydrates, fats and proteins) and micronutrients (vitamins and minerals).

There is international consensus on what constitutes a healthy diet and the 'eatwell plate' (Figure 8.4, Resource 25) provides a pictorial guide for consumers. It shows the different types of food we need to eat – and in what proportions – to have a well-balanced and healthy diet. Advice based on the the 'eatwell plate' will ensure that none of the important nutrients are omitted from the overall diet (for more on ensuring the nutritional adequacy of the diet, see Chapter 8).

Guidance to 'eat healthily' and/or 'have regular meals' rarely achieves weight loss on its own. Extra attention needs to be paid to how to achieve the necessary calorie reduction.
NB There needs to be a daily energy deficit of 600 calories from current energy requirements in order to lose 0.5 kg of body weight per week.

How to use the 'eatwell plate' to achieve an energy deficit

Focus on the FAT of foods eaten:
Frequency
Amount
Type

Frequency

One useful way of helping people to think about how often they eat certain foods is to use the 'eatwell plate' to self-monitor their intake from the different food groups. This helps people to see at a glance how the frequency of consumption is affecting

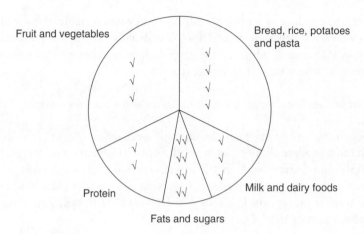

Figure 7.1 Using the 'eatwell plate' to self-monitor frequency of intake from different food groups. Based on the eatwell plate (Department of Health).

the overall balance of the diet. It is then possible to work towards changing the proportions of foods in their diet to be similar to the 'eatwell plate' (Figure 8.4, page 146). Patients can be provided with a **blank plate model** (Tool 5) and asked every time a food is eaten to put a tick in the food group to which it belongs (Figure 7.1 has been filled in for Diary 2).

Patients can see at a glance where proportions need to be altered. In this example, foods from the 'Fats & Sugars' group are consumed most frequently, and there is room to increase fruit and vegetables and starchy foods to resemble the 'eatwell plate'. The patient can still consume favourite foods, but should reduce the **frequency of high-calorie foods** to achieve a calorie deficit. The examples below show how cutting down on how often certain foods are eaten can make substantial calorie savings.

Examples of saving calories by reducing frequency of foods eaten

50 g bar of chocolate (240 kcals)×2 per day = 480 kcals
Chocolate digestive biscuits (83 kcals)×6 per day = 498 kcals
Chips from chip shop (956 kcals)×5 nights = 4780 kcals

Reduce to:

50 g bar of chocolate×1 per day = 240 kcals saved
Chocolate digestive biscuits×2 per day = 332 kcals saved
Chips from chip shop×2 nights = 1912 kcals per week = 273 kcals per day

---

Amount

Developing an awareness of suitable portion sizes is a really important way of cutting down on calories. Over the last few decades, serving sizes of food and drinks, both at home and when eating out, have increased substantially. For some people this is a key cause of their obesity. There are a number of initial steps that can immediately reduce the **amount** of food and drinks consumed, as well as other measures which require a bit more effort. It is usually helpful for patients to make a few changes at a time, which can then be built on, although this will depend to some extent on where they are starting from.

In order to proceed in a stepwise manner to improve portion control:

Take stock of the size of plates, dishes and glasses used
Although most modern dinner plates are the same 10 diameter as 50 years ago, the changes in design often result in the modern version having a reduced rim and therefore a larger area to fill with food. Changing to a smaller plate has been shown to reduce food consumption [5]. This is also the case with tall, slim glasses, which hold smaller volumes than short, wide glasses [4].

Look at food proportions on the plate
A useful visual resource is 'The Healthy Portion Plate' (Resource 16), which shows how much of the plate should be taken up by different foods at lunch and evening meals (Figure 7.2).

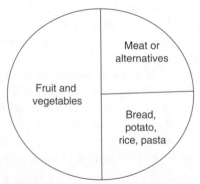

Figure 7.2 Recommended proportions from different food groups at **mealtimes** (the 'eatwell plate' represents the overall balance of the diet). Based on the eatwell plate (Department of Health).

Look at portion sizes of energy-dense foods
Foods such as meat, fish and cheese, as well as the amount of oil, mayonnaise and dressings used, may well make a substantial contribution to a person's calorie intake. They are often sources of 'hidden' calories for someone who is otherwise eating a healthy diet.

Examples of reducing amounts of energy-dense foods eaten

8 oz steak, grilled = 480 kcals	Reduce to: 4 oz steak, grilled = 240 kcals	Saves: 240 kcals
2 oz cheddar cheese = 246 kcals	Reduce to: 1 oz cheddar cheese = 123 kcals	Saves: 123 kcals
2 tbsp olive oil = 258 kcals	Reduce to: 1 tbsp = 129 kcals	Saves: 129 kcals

Establish current portion sizes using a food diary

It may be helpful to ask patients to specifically record the **amounts** of food and drinks consumed. This requires the use of an accurate kitchen scale. It is well recognised that estimating the quantities of a food eaten is difficult as some people have limited understanding of the weights or portions of common foods. This inaccuracy in estimating amounts eaten may partly explain the underestimation of total calories eaten. By concentrating on reducing the **amount** of foods already eaten, the patient can continue to enjoy their preferred foods, and this may help with adherence. A food atlas showing pictures of portion sizes or calorie-counting booklets or apps for smart phones can be very useful visual tools and demonstrate the extent of calorie savings that can be achieved (see Resources 17–20).

Diary 3: patient recording frequency and amount eaten (portion size)

8:00 am	Mug of tea (350 ml) with 40 ml of milk
8:15 am	½ thick-cut slice of white-bread toast (22 g), 1 heaped teaspoon of spread (10 g) & 1 heaped tablespoon of jam (20 g)
9:00 am	Mug of coffee (350 ml) with 40 ml of milk & 2 chocolate sweets from office tin (10 g each)
10:00 am	Mug of coffee (350 ml) with 40 ml of milk & 2 biscuits (17 g each)
12:30 pm	2 thick-cut slices of white bread (44 g each), 1 heaped teaspoon of spread (10 g), 1 heaped tablespoon of mayonnaise (20 g), 1 large egg (50 g) & 1 x 250 ml carton of fruit juice
1:30 pm	½ chocolate bar (24 g)
3:00 pm	Mug of coffee (350 ml) with 40 ml of milk & 1 slice lemon cake (26 g)
5:00 pm	1 apple (133 g)
6:00 pm	Chunk of cheese (57 g)
7:00 pm	1 chicken breast (168 g), 200 g of frozen vegetables, 2 average-sized potatoes (250 g)
7.30 pm	1 yogurt (150 g)
8:00 pm	1 bag of crisps (34.5 g), 1 glass of wine (190 ml)
9:30 pm	Bar of chocolate (49 g)
10:00 pm	Mug of tea (350 ml) with 40 ml of milk

*Estimated calorie content: 2800 kcals

Providing specific individualised portion sizes required for weight loss to individuals requires some calculations to determine total energy requirements for weight loss. This figure can then be converted into specific portions from each food group and is referred to as the 600 kcal deficit diet. Every patient will have different energy needs depending on their age, gender, weight and muscle mass. The heavier the patient, the higher their calorie requirement will be. Appendix 10 provides a formula for estimating individual energy requirements.

An area of confusion…

People get confused with the difference between **portion** sizes and **serving** sizes. Portion sizes refer to portions from the different food groups and are used with the 'eatwell plate' to ensure nutritional adequacy of the diet. Guidance on portion sizes based on the the 'eatwell plate', which will help patients ensure the **nutritional adequacy** of their diet, is provided in Chapter 8.

Serving sizes are what a person eats at one sitting/meal. See the example **serving sizes** for 1500 and 1800 calorie meal plans in Chapter 8 (pages 147 and 148).

Portion control is challenging and often needs to be revisited many times before people really understand how to integrate it into their everyday eating. Supporting patients to become more accurate with their diary-keeping and following the steps outlined above will help to develop the skills necessary to control portions.

Type

Focusing on the types of foods eaten involves changing to lower-calorie versions of particular foods, for example changing from full-cream milk to skimmed or semi-skimmed milk, or from ordinary butter or margarine to half-fat varieties. It is often helpful for patients to learn how to check labels to ensure any nutrition-related claims on the front of packets will genuinely lead to calorie savings.

Diary 4: patient recording frequency, amount and type (FAT)

8:00 am	Mug of tea (350 ml) with 40 ml of full-fat milk
8:15 am	½ thick-cut slice of white-bread toast (22 g), 1 heaped teaspoon of butter (10 g) & 1 heaped tablespoon of jam (20 g)
9:00 am	Mug of coffee (350 ml) with 40 ml of full-fat milk & 2 chocolate sweets from office tin (10 g each)
10:00 am	Mug of coffee with 1/16 with 40 ml of full fat milk & 2 chocolate-coated biscuits (36 g)
12:30 pm	2 thick-cut slices of white bread (44 g), 1 heaped teaspoon of butter (10 g), 1 heaped tablespoon of full-fat mayonnaise (20 g), 1 large egg (50 g) & 1 × 250 ml carton fruit juice
1:30 pm	½ chocolate bar (28 g)
3:00 pm	Mug of coffee (350 ml) with 40 ml of full-fat milk & 1 slice of lemon cake (26 g)
5:00 pm	1 apple (133 g)
6:00 pm	Chunk of mature cheddar cheese (57 g)
7:00 pm	1 skinless chicken breast (168 g) roasted, 200 g of frozen vegetables boiled, 2 average-sized potatoes with skin (250 g) boiled
7:30 pm	1 corner yogurt (150 g)
8:00 pm	1 bag of crisps (34.5 g), 1 glass of red wine (190 ml)
9:30 pm	1 chocolate bar (49 g)
10:00 pm	Mug of tea (350 ml) with 40 ml of full-fat milk

*Estimated calorie content: 3000 kcals

Examples of changing the types of foods eaten

1 pint of full-cream milk = 379 kcals	1 pint semi-skimmed milk = 264 kcals	1 pint skimmed milk = 184 kcals
2 oz cheddar cheese = 206 kcals	2 oz reduced-fat cheddar cheese = 136 kcals	Saves 70 kcals
2 tsp margarine = 100 kcals	2 tsp half-fat margarine = 50 kcals	Saves 50 kcals

How to read the calorie content on labels

Many people use prepackaged convenience foods as part of their everyday diet and it is important that they understand how to interpret food labels. This will allow increased awareness of the calories from each food item. This is essential to weight management in the same way that seeing the price of an item before buying is essential to managing a budget. Currently there are different systems of labelling, which makes the task of understanding more challenging. Chapter 8 describes in detail how to read and understand the different nutrition aspects of a label.

For weight management, it is the calorie content of the food that matters!

A calorie is a calorie whether it comes from protein, fat, carbohydrate or alcohol. Anything eaten in excess leads to weight gain. Weight loss occurs by eating fewer calories than the body needs each day. Some foods are more energy dense than others. The nutrients which provide calories are:

Protein	4 calories per gram
Fat	9 calories per gram
Carbohydrate	4 calories per gram
Alcohol	7 calories per gram

The body needs a combination of foods for health, as outlined in the 'eatwell plate'. One of the common pitfalls is interpreting a product labelled low-fat or low-sugar as meaning calorie-free with no limitation on amounts consumed.

The fat and sugar content of foods matters, but it's *calories that count!*

How to make sense of labels

Foods bought in bulk (e.g. 200 g cheese, 1 litre milk, 500 g meat): individual portions need to be measured at home.
   Tip: For these foods, look at **calories per 100 g** and choose lower-calorie options.
   Ready meals: look for healthy options, which are usually lower in calories.
   Tip: Check for **number of servings per pack** and **calories per serving**.
   Keep to the serving sizes recommended on the pack for bread, cereals, yogurts, desserts, biscuits, cakes and crisps.
   Tip: Get to know 'best value' for calorie foods and stick with the same brands.

Keeping a daily record

Health professionals can be reluctant to ask patients to record calorie intake. However, self-monitoring is known to improve weight-loss success and focusing on calories consumed is crucial to understanding where excess calories are coming from [6].

For those who are struggling to lose weight, this may be a very effective tool. Although many people believe they know about the calorie content of foods, and indeed some are very knowledgeable, in reality many people have a limited understanding. The process of recording calorie intake can help patients learn more about which foods are high and low in calories, allowing informed decisions about food choices. The practice of writing food calories in a diary may alter eating habits as self-awareness increases. It can also allow some flexibility, rather than rigid restraint, as calories can be saved and banked in the run up to special occasions and/or additional savings can be made after an event to compensate for overconsumption.

As self-monitoring calories can be time-consuming, and at times challenging, it is important not to ask patients to keep a diary unnecessarily. For those who are managing their weight well, diary-keeping may be unnecessary (although for some it may be the reason they are coping so well). In some instances it may be helpful to reserve this task for times when patients are struggling to lose weight or when weight loss has plateaued. Learning how to keep a diary accurately is a skill which takes time and its purpose is always for the patient to increase their self-awareness of intake rather than for the health practitioner to check up on their food choices. It helps to explain the purpose of diary-keeping to the patient, as their preconception, or previous experiences of this strategy, may lead to fears of negative, judgmental comments.

'I had no idea how much I was eating until I started to record calories!'

'I have become much more aware of where the hidden calories are in foods, e.g. sandwiches with mayo.'

Diary 5: patient recording frequency, amount, type and calories (kcals)

8:00 am	Mug of tea (350 ml) with 40 ml of full-fat milk, 26 kcals
8:15 am	½ thick-cut slice of white-bread toast (17 g), 45 kcals, 1 heaped teaspoon of butter (10 g), 74 kcals & 1 heaped tablespoon of jam (20 g), 53 kcals
9:00 am	Mug of coffee (350 ml) with 40 ml of full-fat milk, 26 kcals & 2 chocolate sweets (10 g each), 46 kcals & 2 chocolate-coated sweets from the office tin (10 g each), 46 kcals
10:00 am	Mug of coffee (350 ml) with 40 ml of full-fat milk, 23 kcals & 2 chocolate-coated biscuits (36 g) 177 kcals
12:30 pm	2 thick-cut slices of white bread (44 g each), 192 kcals, 1 heaped teaspoon of butter (10 g) 74 kcals, 1 heaped tablespoon of full-fat mayonnaise (20 g) 138 kcals, 1 large egg (50 g) 76 kcals & 1×250 ml carton fruit juice, 93 kcals
1:30 pm	½ chocolate bar (28 g), 140 kcals
3:00 pm	Mug of coffee (350 ml) with 40 ml of full-fat milk, 26 kcals & 1 slice of lemon cake (26 g) 92 kcals
5:00 pm	1 apple (133 g), 60 kcals
6:00 pm	Chunk of mature cheddar cheese (57 g), 273 kcals
7:00 pm	1 skinless chicken breast (168 g) roasted, 239 kcals, 200 g bag of frozen vegetables boiled, 84 kcals, 2 average-sized potatoes with skin (250 g) boiled, 188 kcals
7:30 pm	1 corner yogurt (150 g), 135 kcals
8:00 pm	1 bag of crisps (34.5 g), 186 kcals, 1 glass of red wine (190 ml), 129 kcals
9:30 pm	1 chocolate bar (49 g), 255 kcals
10:00 pm	Mug of tea (350 ml) with 40 ml of full-fat milk, 26 kcals

*Estimated calorie content: 3000 kcals

Note on diary examples

The accuracy of the diaries increases as the recording adds frequency, amount and then type of foods eaten. Recording calorie values helps to increase awareness of the contribution different foods make to calorie intake. This demonstrates how initial attempts at diary-keeping can be as much as 60% inaccurate, as described in the literature [25]. Developing accurate food records is a skill that takes time, but is a worthwhile investment in helping patients increase their awareness.

How to keep a daily calorie record

1 Establish the required calorie intake for weight loss (generally most women will lose weight on 1500 calories/day and most men on 1800 calories/day. Those with higher BMIs will lose weight on higher intakes).
2 Establish how recording is going to occur. Some clients prefer to use their own notebook, others prefer preprinted sheets (Tool 6) or booklets (Resource 21). Some may prefer to use computer records or phone apps.
3 Use a reliable calorie counter (see Resources 17–20).
4 'Record everything, forget nothing' is the golden rule of recording calorie intake. Record time, type and amount of food eaten and the calorie content.
5 Record immediately after eating, if possible – it is easy to forget foods eaten later in the day.
6 Always have the food diary close at hand.

Safety: intake should not be reduced below 1200 calories unless under close medical or dietetic supervision.

> 'Research has demonstrated consistently that self-monitoring is associated with improved weight-loss outcomes.'

How to compare calorie intake with weight-loss achieved

Agreed weight-loss targets should be set at the beginning of any weight-loss intervention. This will vary from person to person:

1 Some may start with weight stabilisation – preventing further weight gain and maintaining current weight. This is why weight history is an important part of the assessment, along with an estimate of current calorie requirements
2 Others may have restrictions on their mobility or be taking medications which affect weight, and weight-loss targets need to be adjusted accordingly. Losing 0.5 kg per month may be realistic for some
3 For those who are aiming to lose weight at the recommended rate of 0.5–1 kg per week over a period of 3–6 months, most men (under 85 kg) will lose weight on 1800 calories and most women (under 95 kg) will lose weight on 1500 calories. Those at higher weights will need to have higher intakes (see Appendix 10 on how to estimate energy requirements, or use the charts in Appendix 11)

When weight loss happens

If target weight is achieved:

1   Use affirmations and encouragement for the effort made
2   Encourage the patient to reflect on what has gone well
3   Discuss any difficulties
4   Ensure diet is well balanced and nutritionally adequate (see Chapter 8)
5   Offer the opportunity to discuss any topics from the 'Menu of Options' (see Chapter 8)
6   Remind the patient that adjustment of calorie intake may be necessary as weight continues to decrease
7   Check if diary-keeping is helpful and if the patient wishes to continue with it

When weight loss doesn't happen

If the target has not been met and the patient is aware of why, move on to working through any difficulties in a problem-solving way.

If target weight loss has not been achieved and the patient cannot understand why, this needs to be handled in a skilled and sensitive manner:

1   This is a clear indication of a discrepancy in the patient's perception of calories consumed versus the actual amount consumed
2   This is very understandable – even the most carefully kept diary will only be 80% accurate [4]
3   Encourage the patient to become a calorie 'detective' to uncover these inaccuracies – see examples of the level of detail that may be required earlier in this chapter. Help the patient understand what aspect of diary-keeping needs to become more accurate – recording frequency, amount, type, calorie-counting
4   Adopt a curiosity about where the hidden calories are and work alongside the patient in identifying possible sources
5   Be empathetic to their situation and resist the temptation to interrogate them about the detail of every food. They are probably feeling very disappointed and frustrated and interrogation might exacerbate those feelings
6   Encourage detailed diary-keeping. The secret is in keeping accurate diaries. Patients cannot change if they are not fully aware of what they are eating

---

Example of a conversation when weight-loss targets are not met

Patient: *'I just cannot understand it! I mean, I really have stuck to my diet.'*
Practitioner: *'You sound very disappointed.'*
Patient: *'Yes, well, it just makes you feel that all that effort isn't worth it!'*
Practitioner: *'I can see that you are really frustrated, especially as you feel you tried really hard. This is the tough part of trying to lose weight – when things don't go as you would like. If it is any consolation, you are not the only person to experience this. Lots of people find it takes time to really get the weight coming off.'*

Patient: *'But I feel I am not making progress. What else can I do?'*
Practitioner: *'Would you like me to share what we have found works when people get stuck?'*
Patient: *'Yes, I am so fed up not to have lost anything!'*
Practitioner: *'What we know for sure is that in order for weight to come off, there needs to be an energy deficit between what you are eating and the energy you use each day. Because your weight has stayed the same, that tells us that you are having the right number of calories to maintain your weight. In order for you to lose weight, we need to find that calorie deficit. This is where the detective work starts!'*
Patient: *'How do you mean? I have kept strictly to 1500 calories!'*
Practitioner: *'It seems you are trying really hard. Researchers have found that it is very difficult to accurately record every mouthful that we eat and drink – most of us esti-mate a shortfall of at least 20%. That is why we now encourage people to practise becoming even more accurate with diary-keeping. What do you think about that?'*
Patient: *'A bit of a pain, but if it works, I guess it is worth it!'*
Practitioner: *'Shall we have a look at how accurate it needs to be?'* [see Diary 4 and 5.]

Using all of the strategies outlined above, 'hidden' sources of calories are often identified and offer possible areas for change (e.g. mayonnaise in sandwiches or oil drizzled over salad or large portion sizes of protein foods). They also show how 'swaps' can achieve significant calorie reductions.

When discussing dietary changes, think about the five Ps:

1   Be **Positive** – focus on what **can** be eaten rather than giving lots of negative advice (e.g. '*Don't have…*', '*Avoid…*' , '*You mustn't eat…*')
2   Be **Practical** – make sure any changes fit in with everyday life
3   Ensure the changes are **Palatable** – include favourite foods
4   Any changes need to be **Possible** – help patients set achievable goals
5   **Personable** – ensure that any suggested changes fit in with personal preferences

Encourage healthy eating as a way of life.

When to refer on to specialist services

If the approaches described above have been tried without success, consider a referral to a Registered Dietitian or person who has received appropriate training in estimating energy requirements and developing an individual eating plan based on these figures. Dietetic services will generally have locally published guidelines on patients who are suitable for referral. This often includes patients who have a BMI above 30 if they have tried first-line treatment and target weight loss has not been achieved, and/or those patients with lower BMIs but other associated conditions which complicate their nutritional management, such as diabetes, CHD or PCOS, as well as those already on a therapeutic diet for an established medical condition such as coeliac disease. Local pathways will also provide guidance on when to refer to multidisciplinary specialist teams.

Further dietary options

Meal replacements

These provide approximately 1200–1600 kcals per day and can work well 'for people who have difficulty with self-selection and/or portion control' [7]. There is sufficient evidence to support the inclusion of meal-replacement approaches as one of a range of possible dietary treatments for the management of overweight and obesity [8]. Meal replacements replace two meals – usually breakfast and lunch – with a shake, soup or bar, and include a 600 calorie healthy meal in the evening. Most plans also allow two to three 100 calorie snacks a day and recommend drinking six to eight glasses of water or low-calorie drinks. They should not be confused with very-low-calorie diets (VLCDs), which provide less than 800 kcal/day.

'I was surprised to learn that meal replacements are an effective evidence-based option.'

Very-low-calorie diets

VLCDs provide less than 800 kcal/day and should only be used under close medical and dietary supervision by experienced and well-qualified health professionals [8].

Popular diets

High-protein/low-carbohydrate
Recent research has shown this approach may suit some individuals during the weight-loss phase of treatment, although its longer term effects remain unclear. This approach needs to be carefully supervised as there is a risk of nutritional inadequacies, and additional support is important during the reintroduction of carbohydrates to minimise weight regain.

Low-glycaemic-index
Although this approach promotes a number of healthy components of the diet, there is little evidence to suggest it is effective for weight loss per se, its role in weight management remains unclear.
For more on evidence-based dietary options, see Chapter 3.

Fad diets
Health care professionals and their patients will be familiar with the many 'fad diets' that are promoted as offering a quick fix for weight loss. People can often be tempted by the lure of 'the magic wand'. It is important to offer evidence-based guidance to those who seek advice about 'fad diets'. The following recommendations from the British Dietetic Association may be helpful to patients in understanding how to spot a fad diet [9]:

It's a fad diet if it ...

- recommends strange quantities of only one food, e.g. grapefruit, meat, eggs, cabbage
- promotes magical foods to 'burn' fats
- suggests rigid menus, limiting food choice
- advises food should only be eaten in certain combinations
- suggests rapid weight loss of more than 1 kg per week
- doesn't address barriers to losing weight
- fails to recommend physical activity
- doesn't advise people with medical conditions to seek medical advice before starting

Conclusion

Putting dietary recommendations into practice is a huge challenge for patients in today's obesogenic environment. Practitioners need to be fully informed and aware of how difficult this can be. They need to work collaboratively with patients to overcome these challenges in order to move towards successful and rewarding outcomes.

Consider this

1 What advice do you currently give about diet?
2 Is the advice in line with current dietary guidelines?
3 Is the advice tailored to the individual?
4 Do you feel equipped to help patients develop self-awareness regarding their eating and activity habits?
5 Do you listen empathically to patients who struggle and help them explore different options until they find solutions?
6 What resources do you use?

Recommendations for physical activity

It is widely recognised that physical activity is important to risk reduction for chronic disease and improved overall health. Studies show a 30% decrease in all-cause mortality and a substantial impact on the risk of coronary heart disease, stroke, hypertension, type 2 diabetes, chronic renal disease and some cancers. Activity is also known to have a positive impact on osteoporosis, back pain and osteoarthritis and to reduce the risk of depression and anxiety and promote positive mental health and self-esteem. It promotes better independence later in life, improves sleep and creates a sense of achievement and enjoyment. Despite the multiple health gains associated with being physically active, only 42% of men and 31% of women meet the physical-activity recommendations for health [10]. Interestingly, 80% of adults perceive themselves to be physically active. In addition to the many health benefits associated with increased activity, there are some specific benefits particularly relevant to weight management:

1   Helps prevent overweight and obesity
2   Helps reduce weight effectively when combined with a reduced energy intake
3   Helps with weight maintenance and prevention of weight regain

Inactivity contributes to 35000 deaths per year.

Current physical activity guidelines for *all* adults

1   Adults should aim to be active daily. Activity should add up to *at least* **150 minutes per week of moderate-intensity activity** in bouts of 10 minutes or more – one way to approach this is to do 30 minutes on at least 5 days a week [12,13]
2   Alternatively, comparable benefits can be achieved through 75 minutes of vigorous-intensity activity spread across the week or a combination of moderate- and vigorous-intensity activity [12,13]
3   Adults should also undertake physical activity to improve muscle strength on at least 2 days a week [12,13]
4   All adults should minimise the amount of time spent being sedentary (sitting) for extended periods [12,13]

Recommendations for weight management

1   Reducing inactivity should be a component of weight-management programmes [2,3]
2   Overweight and obese individuals should be supported to undertake increased physical activity as part of a multicomponent weight-management programme [2,3]
3   Overweight and obese individuals should be prescribed a volume of physical activity equal to approximately 1800–2500 kcal/week. This corresponds to

approximately **225–300 minutes/week** of **moderate-intensity** physical activity (which may be achieved through **five sessions** of **45–60 minutes** per week, or lesser amounts of vigorous physical activity). This can be achieved in several short bursts of 10 minutes or more [3]

4   People who have lost weight may need to do **60–90 minutes** on 5 or more days per week to avoid regaining weight [2]

First steps towards achieving physical-activity recommendations for weight management

Safety: It is important to ensure that individuals have no contraindications to exercise before commencing a physical-activity programme. The Physical Activity Readiness Questionnaire (PAR-Q) [3] (Appendix 9) and the General Practice Physical Activity Questionnaire (GPPAQ) [13] (Appendix 8) are quick and validated tools for determining whether additional assessment and investigations are required prior to embarking on increased physical activity.

Step1: reduce sedentary behaviours

Limit screen time (TV, computers, games consoles)
- Increase any movement
- Avoid sitting for longer than half an hour – move around

Step 2: build up gradually

- Start with establishing current levels of activity and build daily activity from there

Step 3: move on to increasing daily activity and include some structured activities

- Tailor to individual preferences
- Include everyday activities (housework, gardening, etc.)
- Consider walking schemes and group activities
- Be aware of local leisure service facilities

Step 4: consider guidance on muscle-strengthening exercise

- Resistance training is the most effective method available for maintaining and increasing lean body mass and improving muscular strength and endurance [13]
- Refer to physical-activity specialists for advice on resistance training

Step 5: encourage activity as a way of life – essential for maintenance of weight lost

- Consider referral to an exercise specialist for individual advice

Practical application of physical-activity recommendations

Promoting physical activity

How does physical activity help?

1 Increases total energy expenditure.
2 Promotes body fat metabolism while preserving lean mass.
3 Increases metabolic rate.

The challenge for the practitioner is to create awareness and understanding of physical activity messages and to facilitate engagement and participation in increased levels of activity.

What gets in the way?

Barriers to activity

- lack of knowledge of the benefits
- lack of time
- lack of someone to exercise with
- not being 'the sporty type'
- financial constraints
- lack of suitable facilities
- lack of 'willpower'
- fear of embarrassment
- lack of enjoyment
- Fear of overdoing it, resulting in injury

Addressing barriers to being more active

1 Barriers to activity (whether real or perceived) need to be understood and addressed in an empathic manner
2 Practitioners can play a key role in providing information in a helpful way, addressing concerns and problem-solving with the patient to find a way of becoming more active
3 Information can be provided on the benefits of being more active in a helpful way
4 Practitioners can build and strengthen motivation by actively listening and reflecting concerns
5 Progress should be reviewed at each appointment

Where to start?

Step 1: reducing inactivity
Often, the first step is to focus on reducing inactivity. It can be useful to ask patients to record hours of inactivity in order to raise awareness (see Figure 7.3, Tool 3).

Time in hours

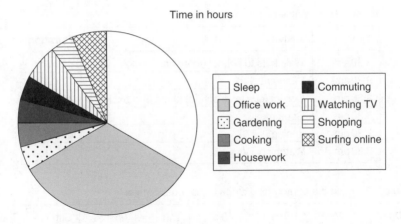

Figure 7.3   Time spent on different activities over 24 hours.

Once a pattern becomes clear, encourage patients to think about **how** they can reduce inactivity. Be careful not to make suggestions uninvited – '*Why don't you...*' Instead encourage patients to come up with their own ideas, and if appropriate, discuss some of the ideas below: '*Shall we look at some ideas that others have suggested?*' Help patients develop a Change Plan around reducing inactivity (see Tool 4).

Ideas for reducing inactivity

- Reduce screen time (TV/computers/games consoles)
- Stand rather than sit
- Take a break from sitting every half hour
- Hide the remote control
- Don't leave items at the bottom of the stairs – make the journey each time
- Walk around when talking on the phone
- Walk to the newsagent/post box/local shops
- Don't ask other people to run errands – do it yourself!
- Climb the stairs more often – at home and instead of using a lift
- Make activity part of social life, e.g. meet friends for 'walk and talk'
- Get off the bus a stop earlier
- Park the car further away from the office/supermarket
- Offer to take a neighbour's dog for a walk
- Walk with children to and from school
- Have 'walking' meetings at work

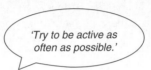

'*Try to be active as often as possible.*'

Steps 2 & 3: increasing daily activity
Increasing activity is essential for supporting weight loss **and** maintaining this loss over time. Help patients become more aware of their current levels of activity

Table 7.1   Example of an activity diary

Time	Activity	Duration
8.30 am	Walk kids to school (there and back)	40 mins
9.30 am	Sitting at work	
3.30 pm	Collect kids from school (there and back)	40 mins
5.30 pm	Cook meal	30 mins
7.30 pm	Ironing	60 mins
8.30 pm	Watching TV	

Table 7.2   Example of recording steps using a pedometer

Day	Mon	Tue	Wed	Thu	Fri	Sat	Sun
Steps	3439	3571	4925	3564	3750	5179	3423

through **diary-keeping** (Table 7.1) or wearing a **pedometer** (Table 7.2). The next step is to gradually build up levels of activity until they have reached the recommended levels for weight loss and maintenance. This takes time and needs to be revisited at each consultation.

During weight-loss phase, aim to increase activity to:

- **45–60 minutes 5 times per week of moderate-intensity activity**   This will contribute 1800–2500 calories per week (3500 calories is approximately equivalent to 0.5 kg of body fat), emphasising the importance of combining activity with dietary changes to achieve the desired weight-loss outcome of 0.5–1 kg /week.

During weight-maintenance phase, aim for:

- **60–90 minutes 5 times per week of moderate-intensity activity**   A person who has lost weight is susceptible to weight regain and maintaining a high level of activity helps to sustain increased lean body mass. The impact on metabolism helps to sustain the weight lost (this would contribute 2400–3600 calories to energy expenditure, allowing for adjustment of food intake).

In practical terms: as these levels can be daunting for those who are inactive, it may be more helpful to talk to patients about becoming an 'active person', with the aim of achieving a level of activity that will help support weight maintenance. People who start from a very inactive lifestyle may take some time to reach the optimal levels of activity, so the overall health benefits need to be emphasised, along with the message that 'every calorie counts' and the importance of paying attention to **calorie intake** as well as **calorie output**.

What does *moderate-intensity activity* feel like?

- Breathing and heartbeat a little faster than usual. It should still be possible to have a conversation, but not sing
- It feels warm and the person may sweat

It is important to find an activity the individual enjoys as they are much more likely to sustain such changes. It is helpful to be well informed about the range of physical-activity options in your area and to support patients in developing a change plan for increasing activity.

Range of activities

- walking (individually or in groups)
- cycling
- gardening
- swimming
- going to the gym
- dancing
- playing a sport, e.g. badminton, football or bowls
- stretching exercise, e.g. yoga or Pilates
- housework
- playing in the garden

Table 7.3 Intensities and energy expenditures for common types of physical activity (Department of Health [12])

Activity	Intensity	Intensity (METs)	Energy expenditure (kcal equivalent, for a person of 60 kg doing the activity for 30 minutes)
Ironing	Light	2.3	69
Cleaning and dusting	Light	2.5	75
Walking – strolling, 2 mph	Light	2.5	75
Painting/decorating	Moderate	3.0	90
Walking – 3 mph	Moderate	3.3	99
Hoovering	Moderate	3.5	105
Golf – walking, pulling clubs	Moderate	4.3	129
Badminton – social	Moderate	4.5	135
Tennis – doubles	Moderate	5.0	150
Walking – brisk, 4 mph	Moderate	5.0	150
Mowing the lawn – walking, power-mower	Moderate	5.5	165
Cycling – 10–12 mph	Moderate	6.0	180
Aerobic dancing	Vigorous	6.5	195
Cycling – 12–14 mph	Vigorous	8.0	240
Swimming – slow crawl, 50 yards/minute	Vigorous	8.0	240
Tennis – singles	Vigorous	8.0	240
Running – 6 mph (10 minutes/mile)	Vigorous	10.0	300
Running – 7 mph (8.5 minutes/mile)	Vigorous	11.5	345
Running – 8 mph (7.5 minutes/mile)	Vigorous	13.5	405

MET = metabolic equivalent. 1 MET = a person's metabolic rate (of energy expenditure) when at rest; 2 METs = a doubling of the resting metabolic rate.

Sometimes people become disheartened when they see how many calories they burn from what feels like a great deal of hard work (see Table 7.3). It is important to convey the message that 'every calorie counts', especially when the activity is undertaken daily. Increasing activity alone rarely achieves weight loss, which is why paying attention to food intake is so important. Building activity during the weight-loss phase of treatment really pays off in helping to sustain weight lost.

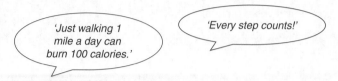

'Just walking 1 mile a day can burn 100 calories.'

'Every step counts!'

Encourage patients to become 'an active person' for life

Getting started

1   Raise the issue of activity as part of a weight-management intervention
2   Screen for safety and current level of activity using GPPAQ or PAR-Q
3   Intervene:
    i.   provide nonjudgmental feedback on GPPAQ classification
    ii.   provide information on recommended levels of activity for weight management
    iii.   check for engagement by asking *'Are you happy to explore ways of increasing your activity?'*
    iv.   explore options, e.g. wear a pedometer, refer on to local physical activity specialists or schemes like 'Walking for Health'
    v.   develop a change plan around increasing activity
4   Review at each appointment

Then, under supervision of a qualified instructor:
Aim to achieve a combination of increased daily activity: some structured activities 2–3 times a week, including muscle-strengthening exercises [11].

Wearing a pedometer
Many people find it difficult to fit activity into their daily lives. Researchers have found that people who increase their activity throughout the day can achieve the same health benefits as people who are sedentary for most of the day and go to the gym for half an hour.

How many steps?

- 10 000 steps a day is the recommended target
- 10 000 steps = 4–5 miles
- 2000 steps = 1 mile
- 1 mile = approx. 100 calories

Steps per minute of activity:

Slow walking:	100 steps/minute
Moderate walking:	110 steps/minute
Fast walking:	125+ steps/minute

Getting started with a pedometer

- Put it on first thing in the morning and wear until bedtime – ensure it is worn correctly
- Wear for 7 days to establish baseline, e.g. a weekly total of 31 500 steps = 4500 per day
- Increase by 500 steps per day and when that is established add another 500 steps per day
- Remember the target is 10 000 steps per day or more
- The practitioner should encourage the use of pedometers by wearing one themself!

'In 5 minutes you can add 500 steps to your day!'

'A person who walks 10 000 steps/day will burn 2000–3500 calories per week!'

For those who do not wish to use a pedometer

Examples of moderate-intensity-activity equivalents of 10 000 steps a day

- Washing windows or floors for 45–60 minutes
- Gardening for 45–60 minutes
- Brisk walking for 30 minutes (ideally 2 miles)
- Cycling 5 miles in 30 minutes
- Ballroom dancing for 30 minutes
- Raking leaves for 30 minutes
- Swimming lengths for 20 minutes

Consider this

- Do you currently include discussions about activity in all your weight-management consultations?
- Are you doing enough to promote activity?
- What else can you do?
- What services are available in your area?

Developing essential skills: laying the foundations

Besides being equipped with essential knowledge on eating and activity, patients need to become skilled at managing their eating and activity in a variety of situations lifelong. Although there are a wide range of skills required in the initial stages of a weight-management programme, the key ones:

1   problem-solving (covered earlier in this chapter)
2   self-monitoring
3   goal-setting.

Further skills will need to be developed as the intervention progresses, and these are covered in more detail in Chapters 8 and 9.

Self-monitoring

Continuing to build a picture

Completing an assessment (Chapter 6) helps gain an initial picture and identify difficulties, which can then be explored before moving on to find solutions. The nature of change means that building a picture needs to be an ongoing process and self-monitoring helps to achieve this.

Keeping a diary

Keeping a diary is recognised as a key behavioural tool for weight management [6]. Its purpose is to help the patient become more aware of current behaviours and identify problem areas. Solutions can then be explored and decided upon using the steps of the problem-solving process outlined earlier in this chapter. Diary-keeping needs to be tailored to the individual in order to ensure they gain maximum benefit from the process. It is not meant to be used as a tool for the practitioner to 'check up on the patient', although patients may perceive this to be the case. As it is such a useful tool, it is important to get it right from the beginning.

What to record?

The content and format may change over time depending on what the patient is working on. Examples include:

1   food intake
2   activity
3   body weight
4   personal achievements
5   new skills acquired
6   comments.

Table 7.4   Detailed food diary

Time	Food and Amount	*Calories	Place	Comment
7.30 am	30 g cornflakes 200 ml semi-skimmed milk 1 cup tea & 30 ml milk	112 100 15	Home	In a rush
10 am	Coffee (no sugar) & 100 ml semi-skimmed milk 95 g banana	– 50 90	Work	Said no to biscuits!
12.30 pm	2 slices wholemeal bread (100 g) 3 oz chicken & salad 10 g low-fat mayo 100 g apple & 80 g satsuma	108 126 30 50 + 21	Work Common Room	Made sandwich myself
3 pm	60 g chocolate cake	283	Home	Felt peckish
7 pm	120 g roast lamb 4 tbsp vegetables 200 g potato	248 17 + 17 143	Home	Ate with partner
8 pm	120 g yogurt	75	Watching TV	Felt like something sweet
9 pm	Tea & 30 ml milk	15		No biscuits!
	Total Calories	**1500**		

Comments: Not a bad day. I could have had a smaller piece of cake. Need to get rid of the crisps – too tempting! Keep going!

Food intake

Research shows most people initially underestimate their food intake and accuracy increases as the recording period increases. The more accurate participants become in recording their food intake, the more successful they are likely to be at losing weight. It is a skill that is worth building, but it takes time and requires practice. It may be helpful for patients to gradually build up the skill of keeping a diary, starting with simple records and then moving on to more detailed and complex diaries. Examples of food diaries can be found throughout this chapter, and an even more detailed diary is given in Table 7.4.

Note: We have not included diary examples of 'Food, Mood and Thoughts' as interpretation of these requires expertise beyond the scope of this book. It begins to move into the field of cognitive behavioural therapy, which requires the skills of an appropriately trained therapist working under supervision. This support can be offered by specialist services. 'Overcoming Weight Problems' is an excellent self-help resource for those patients who wish to explore this topic further (Resource 22).

Activity

People tend to overestimate their activity level and keeping a record helps patients become more aware of their actual activity levels and highlights opportunities for increasing activity and decreasing inactivity.

Example of a patient's recording activity

Recording steps

	Mon	Tue	Wed	Thu	Fri	Sat	Sun
Steps	3439	3571	4925	3564	3750	5179	3423

Recording minutes of activity

	Mon	Tue	Wed	Thu	Fri	Sat	Sun
Activity	Cleaning	Cinema	Cooking	Cooking	Cooking	Cleaning	Gardening
Time	30 mins	–	30 mins	30 mins	30 mins	2 hours	2 hours

Body weight

People who lose weight and keep it off long-term are more likely to weigh themselves regularly. During the weight-loss phase, it helps track progress and provides
feedback for the patient on the impact of eating and activity changes. Experts
suggest weekly weighing, or more recently, daily weighing. Health care professionals often express concerns that regular weighing may increase the tendency to over-
focus on weight changes. However, despite these concerns, regular weighing seems
to help patients register that fluctuations in body weight are normal and identify
early any changes in the weight trend (Tool 7). Table 7.5 shows an example of
a weekly weight chart.

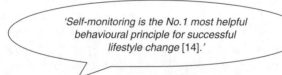

'Self-monitoring is the No.1 most helpful
behavioural principle for successful
lifestyle change [14].'

Personal achievements

Although people respond well to encouragement from others, they can also benefit
from encouragement from themselves. A very effective way of doing this is through
the use of a diary – using stars, smiley faces or words of encouragement.

New skills acquired

Diaries can be used to track new skills such as eating more slowly, or for recording
and recognising changes in hunger scores (see Chapter 8).

Comments

Diaries can be used to make personal observations or comments on progress and
practitioners should encourage patients to make sense and interpret what they record.

Diaries are very personal records and need to be respected as such. People may
find it difficult to keep accurate records, especially initially, when they are practising

Table 7.5 Weekly weight chart

Weight	Week 1	Week 2	Week 3	Week 4	Week 5	Week 6	Week 7	Week 8	Week 9	Week 10	Week 11	Week 12
13st 7	●											
13st 6												
13st 5												
13st 4		●										
13st 3			●									
13st 2												
13st 1				●								
13st 0												
12st 13					●							
12st 11						●						
12st 10							●					
12st 9								●				
12st 8									●			
12st 7										●		
12st 6												
12st 5											●	
12st 4												●

and learning the skill. Some may find it painful or embarrassing to write down exactly what they have eaten. Encourage people to build the skill, but be mindful that some may not find this easy. Ideally, patients will want to share their records, but if not, encourage them to talk about the experience and what they have learnt, to describe goods days and not-so-good days. Help patients to interpret their records and to act upon those observations.

How long should people keep diaries? For as long as they are helpful! If patients are losing weight without keeping a diary, don't ask them to undertake an unnecessary task. Diaries are useful for patients who are struggling with their weight, and people often find that if they stop keeping records, their weight starts to creep back up. As a behavioural strategy, keeping a diary is invaluable, but it must be tailored to the individual.

Goal-setting

On the whole, patients are surprisingly unskilled in goal-setting. Unrealistic goals set people up for failure. It may be useful to discuss the consequences of previous experiences of setting unrealistic goals.

For a goal to make a difference in the time set to achieve it, it needs to be as far-reaching as possible. For example, if the main goal is to reduce calorie intake, the main dietary source of calorie-dense foods needs to be identified and reduced to a level that will make a difference – the 600 kcal daily deficit.

Only two or three specific, realistic and achievable changes should be chosen at any one time. Once an area of work has been decided on, patients can be encouraged to divide their goals into a series of smaller steps, and as these are reached, they can begin to move towards their larger goal. Successful negotiation of each of the smaller steps gives patients a sense of achievement, keeping them motivated over the longer term.

Once the nature of the goal has been agreed, it can help to explore with the patient how they intend to implement the plan. Patients' intentions can be summarised by completing a **Change Plan** (Tool 4).

Developing a **Change Plan** helps patients achieve **SMART goals** in a practical way.

Example of a Change Plan: food

What change am I going to make?	*'Cut down on portion sizes of meat.'*
How am I going to make sure it happens?	*'At home, weigh the amount of meat on my plate for 1 week.'*
What might get in the way?	*'Eating away from home.'*
How will I get round that?	a) *'Ask for smaller portions.'*
	b) *'Leave some on the plate.'*
When will I start?	*'Tonight.'*

Encourage patients to imagine making the changes. e.g. *'Can you imagine yourself doing that each day?'*

The more detailed the plan, the better!

Conclusion

This chapter has focused on the foundations of successful weight management – taking initial steps towards achieving diet and activity changes, through working with patients in a collaborative way and integrating key behavioural approaches.

Consider this

You have just helped a client develop a plan for weight loss.
Is **the plan**:

S – Specific (What exactly are they going to change?)
M – Measurable (Can the change be measured?)
A – Achievable (Is this plan going to be possible for this client?)
R – Realistic (Are the planned changes realistic and likely to fit in?)
T – Time-specific (When is it going to start?)

If the plan focuses on the **what**, **how** and **when** of change, it should be **SMART**.

Note: *netWISP Nutritional Analysis Package was used for dietary calculations of food diaries appearing in this chapter [15].

References

1. Department of Health. Healthy Weight, Healthy Lives: A Toolkit for Developing Local Strategies. http://www.dh.gov.uk/en/Publicationsandstatistics/Publications/DH_088968; 2008.
2. National Institute for Clinical Excellence. Obesity: Guidance on the Prevention, Identification, Assessment and Management of Overweight and Obesity in Adults and Children. NICE; 2006.
3. Scottish Intercollegiate Guidelines Network. Management of Obesity: A National Clinical Guideline. SIGN; 2010.
4. Wansink B. Mindless Eating: Why We Eat More Than We Think. New York: Bantum Dell; 2006.
5. Wansink B, van Ittersum K. Portion size me: downsizing our consumption norms. J Am Diet Assoc 2007 Jul;107[7]:1103–6.
6. Burke L, Wang J, Sevick M. Self-monitoring in weight loss: a systematic review of the literature Journal of American Dietetics Association 2011;111[1]:92–102.
7. American Dietetic Association Evidence Library. Effectiveness in Terms of Client Adherence and Weight Loss and Maintenance of Meal Replacements; 2006.
8. DOMUK. Position Paper on Meal Replacements. http://www.domuk.org/viewpage.php?cat=8&page=25; 2005.
9. The British Dietetic Association. The Truth About Fad Diet. http://www.bda.uk.com/foodfacts/TruthFadDiets.pdf; 2011.
10. The Information Centre for Health and Social Care. The Health Survey for England. http://www.ic.nhs.uk/statistics-and-data-collections/health-and-lifestyles-related-surveys/health-survey-for-england. NHS; 2008.

11. BHF National Centre for Physical Activity and Health. Physical Activity Guidelines in the UK: Review and Recommendations. Loughborough University; 2010.

12. Department of Health. Start Active, Stay Active. A Report on Physical Activity for Health from the Four Home Countries' Chief Medical Officers. DoH; 2011.

13. National Obesity Observatory. Brief Interventions for Weight Management. http://www.noo.org.uk/uploads/doc/vid_10702_BIV2.pdf; 2011.

14. Foreyt J. Weight Loss: Counseling and Long-term Management: A Physician's Toolbox of Counseling Strategies. http://www.medscape.org/viewarticle/493028; 2010.

15. *netWISP Nutritional Analysis Package. http://www.tinuvielsoftware.com/wisp.htm; 2011.

8 Next Steps: Continuing to Develop Expertise

'To get through the hardest journey we need take only one step at a time, but we must keep on stepping.'

Chinese proverb

Review appointments

Introduction

Once initial steps have been taken and a solid weight-management foundation is in place, the next phase is to continue to build on the knowledge and skills already acquired. Follow-up appointments are an opportunity to review progress. Initially this will relate to progress in putting the foundations in place (Chapter 7) but thereafter it is an opportunity to expand expertise.

Review appointments need to be structured and exactly how this is arranged will depend to some degree on local resources. However, patients should be clear about how review appointments will be organised, as well as the number, duration and frequency of visits. Review appointments can be spread over a 6-month period, initially weekly or biweekly, with each visit requiring a minimum of 10–15 minutes. Flexibility is important though, and if good progress is being made, review appointments can be spread over a longer period.

Suggested structure for review appointments

- Review progress with changes to eating and activity (using a diary). Discuss what has gone well/not so well
  - Affirm success and encourage
  - Discuss any difficulties using reflective listening skills
- Review progress with weight
  - Affirm success and encourage
  - Discuss any difficulties using reflective listening skills

Weight Management: A Practitioner's Guide, First Edition. Dympna Pearson and Clare Grace.
© 2012 Dympna Pearson and Clare Grace. Published 2012 by Blackwell Publishing Ltd.

- Explore options and set new goals, using a Change Plan (Tool 4)
- Discuss support
- Discuss ways of reinforcing new habits (rewards or encouragers)
- Discuss a topic from the 'Menu of Options' (Figures 8.1 and 8.2 and Tools 9 and 10) and/or some strategies or skills for weight management. The next section covers topics which can be discussed at review appointments. The section after that covers skills and strategies that are known to be helpful

Review progress at 3 and 6 months

At 3 months:

- If no progress, consider medication or referral to a specialist unit, depending on BMI
- Consider: 'Is the treatment working?', and if not, discuss appropriate action with the patient

At 6 months:

- Some patients may wish to continue with weight loss and need regular visits for support
- Some may wish to maintain the weight they have lost and still require ongoing support for weight maintenance
- Discuss whether the programme is suitable for the patient and is achieving the agreed targets

If at any stage the patient exits the programme, ensure medical problems receive continuing care and that the patient continues to feel supported regardless of their weight

Review appointments: Checklist for agreement with patient

- ☐ Duration of the weight-loss phase of treatment
- ☐ Frequency of review visits
- ☐ Time allocated for each visit
- ☐ Appointment times for the first month
- ☐ Need for continuous care and support during weight-maintenance phase
- ☐ Review at 3 and 6 months

Topics for review appointments

Menu of Options

Figure 8.1 gives a sample 'Menu of Options' of topics for discussion at review appointments. The blank circles are for topics that the patient may wish to discuss (see also Tool 9).

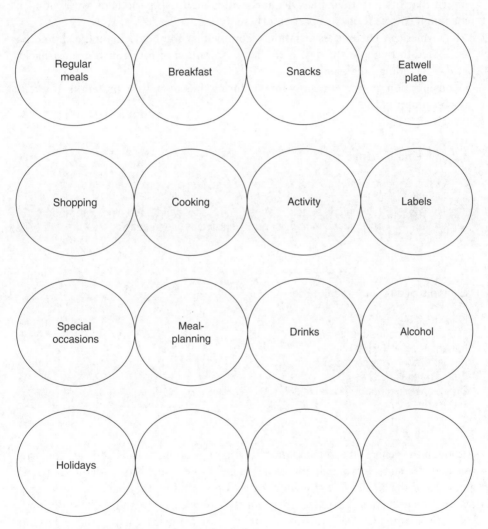

Figure 8.1   Menu of Options – knowledge topics.

Regular meals

'Regardless of meal distribution, a negative energy balance is the most important factor affecting weight loss.'

There is insufficient evidence to make absolute recommendations about meal frequency. Clinical judgment must be used to guide patients towards finding a meal pattern that fits into their lifestyle, and avoids high-risk periods of 'over'-hunger, when high-calorie foods are particularly tempting.

The American Dietetic Association recommends 'Total caloric intake should be distributed throughout the day, with the consumption of four to five meals/snacks per day including breakfast'.

Consumption of greater energy intake during the day may be preferable to evening consumption [1].

Guidance for patients

- Aim for a regular eating pattern, e.g. breakfast, lunch, evening meal
- Avoid going for long periods without food
- Have healthy low-calorie snacks between meals to avoid becoming over-hungry
- Aim for 4–5 hours between meals and 2–3 hours between snacks

---

Example of a regular meal pattern

Breakfast: 7–8 am
Mid-am: tea/coffee and snack
Lunch: 12.30–1.30 pm
Mid-afternoon: tea/coffee and snack
Evening meal: 6–7 pm
During the evening: drink and snack

Although the general recommendation is to avoid skipping meals and eat regularly, this may not suit everyone. If someone struggles to eat small-to-moderate portions at a meal or snack, and finds the more eating opportunities they have, the more they overeat, it's quite possible that eating four to five times a day isn't the best option.

If erratic eating has been identified, often the first step is to help patients develop regular eating patterns. For those with disordered eating, consider the use of a self-help manual [2] (Resource 15), or refer to specialist services when the condition is more serious [3].

Breakfast

When it comes to weight loss, breakfast is an important meal. After a long period without eating, blood sugar levels are likely to be lower and skipping breakfast may increase the chances of food cravings, which may result in snacking on unhealthy foods. Research has shown that those who skip breakfast tend to eat more later in the day and US research on those successful in sustaining weight loss shows regular breakfast eating is common [4].

If someone is not in the habit of eating breakfast, they may find it difficult to start. Comments often include: *'If I eat breakfast, I will be sick,'* or *'if I eat breakfast, I can't stop eating all day!'*

Breakfast doesn't have to be eaten first thing in the morning; it can be consumed within the first couple of hours after getting up. It literally 'breaks the fast' from the evening before.

Example of a discussion about breakfast

Practitioner: *'It sounds as if you are not a breakfast person?'*
Patient: *'No, if I eat breakfast...'*
Practitioner: *'Would you be interested to know more about why breakfast is so strongly recommended?'*
Patient: *'OK.'*
Practitioner: *'People who eat breakfast tend to be more successful at losing weight, and keeping it off too! It seems to stop you from getting over-hungry later in the day and it gets your metabolism working more efficiently right from the start of the day.'*
Patient: *'Mm, what do you suggest?'*

Try to avoid 'you should' or 'you need to' eat breakfast.

Breakfast ideas (250 calories)

- 45 g cereal (3 tablespoons), preferably wholegrain + 100 ml milk, 60 g banana
- 220 g porridge made with milk (4 tablespoons)
- 60 g muesli (2 tablespoons) + 100 ml milk
- 52 g toast (2 slices), preferably wholegrain + 10 g margarine + 10 g jam/marmalade
- 120 g yogurt (1 pot) + fruit (2 portions)
- 2 poached eggs on toast (1 slice) + tomato
- 210 g baked beans on toast (1 slice)
- Grilled mushrooms (4) and bacon (2 slices) on toast (1 slice)

Use minimum amounts of butter, margarine or oil.
NB Check the portion sizes.

Snacks

Patients are often confused about whether to have snacks or not, and if so what types of snacks are suitable. Snacks are a good way of avoiding becoming over-hungry between meals and, so long as they are healthy and low-calorie, they can be included as part of a calorie-controlled diet.

'Total calories consumed throughout the day is what matters most.'

Problems arise when people think of snacks as high-fat, energy-dense foods such as crisps, chocolate, biscuits, cakes and so on. Practitioners need to give clear guidance on the types of snacks suitable and help people incorporate them into their daily food plan.

Example of a discussion about snacks

Practitioner: *'You said you felt there was room to cut back on the snacks?'*
Patient: *'Yes, well, I know I have too many!'*
Practitioner: *'Shall we look at what your preferences are and compare with some lower-calorie options?'*
Patient: *'Yes, I need some idea.'*
[Read labels or use a calorie-counting booklet (see Resources 17–20) to check the calorie content of current snacks. This needs to be done collaboratively.]
Practitioner: *'And here are some ideas for alternatives'* [show the list below or photographs – Resource 17].
Patient: *'Yes, I know fruit would be a better choice, but I fancy a currant bun too!'*
Practitioner: *'If we look at your meal plan for the day, we can see if you can fit them both in.'*

Ideas for snacks (100 calories)

- Fruit (1–2 portions)
- 2 plain biscuits
- 1 slice of malt loaf
- 1 currant bun
- 1 low-fat yogurt (125 g)
- 1 slice of bread and jam
- 2 rice cakes
- 3 tablespoons of cereal

Use minimum amounts of butter, margarine or oil.
NB Check the portion sizes.

Drinks

An adequate intake of fluids is essential for health, and particularly important as part of a weight-loss programme. People may mistake thirst for hunger, so encourage patients to ensure that they are drinking sufficient fluids. Contrary to popular belief, beverages such as tea, coffee and fruit squashes count towards fluid intake.

> **Recommendation**
>
> - Aim to drink six to eight medium glasses of fluid daily (1.5 litres)
> - More fluids may be required if physically active or during hot weather
> - Check if adequately hydrated by urine colour. If a pale straw colour, fluid intake is probably fine, but if dark yellow, fluid intake is probably inadequate

NB Watch out for calorie-laden drinks such as sugar-containing fizzy drinks, mixers, fruit juices and smoothies.

Calorie content of common drinks

Fruit juices – 160 ml glass

Tomato juice	22 kcal
Orange juice	58 kcal
Cranberry juice	98 kcal

Fruit drinks are usually served as **275 ml bottles** = 132 kcal

Smoothies – 250 ml bottle

Range from 103 to 176 kcal per bottle.

Cola Drinks

Full-sugar
160 ml glass = 66 kcal
330 ml can = 142 kcal
500 ml bottle = 210 kcal
1 litre bottle = 435 kcal

Diet cola
330 ml can Diet Coke = 1 kcal

Café latte	Regular (254 ml)	Medium (473 ml)	Large (591 ml)
Skimmed	102 kcal	148 kcal	176 kcal
Semi-skim	131 kcal	188 kcal	223 kcal
Whole	168 kcal	242 kcal	289 kcal

Alcohol

Alcoholic drinks are often high in calories and so must be considered as part of a calorie-controlled diet. Check the patient's favourite drink and give information on the calorie content.

Example of a discussion about alcohol

Practitioner: *'What is your favourite drink?'*
Patient: *'Wine – too much of it!'*
Practitioner: *'Well, you don't have to cut it out completely. It just needs to fit into your overall calorie intake.'*
Patient: *'I honestly can't tell you how much I drink – we just keep a bottle in the fridge.'*
Practitioner: *'Perhaps you can keep a record over the next few weeks to get a better idea. Meanwhile, the recommended amount is 1–2 glasses (pub measures!) per day for overall health. At least if you start writing it down, you will have a better idea.'*
Patient: *'I have been thinking of cutting down for a while anyhow.'*
Practitioner: *'Remember: "willpower dissolves in alcohol"!'*

Calorie content of alcoholic drinks

Drink	kcals (approx.)
1 pint beer	200
1 glass wine	100
1 measure of spirits	70
Liqueurs (50 ml)	170

Drinks	Single	Double
Bacardi & Diet Coke	65 kcal	130 kcal
Bacardi & Coke	129 kcal	194 kcal
Vodka, lime and soda	76 kcal	131 kcal
Vodka & tonic	88 kcal	143 kcal
Gin & slim line tonic	56 kcal	112 kcal
Gin & tonic	120 kcal	175 kcal

It pays to become aware of the calorie content of drinks!

Portion control

Portion sizes have increased over the last couple of decades and this has probably had a significant impact on expanding waistlines. Patients find it difficult to estimate an average portion. As food portions outside the home have increased, so the use of larger plates, serving dishes and glasses has encouraged larger portions at home. In addition, some restaurants offer extra helpings and takeaways offer 'supersizes'. In supermarkets, the trend for 'buy one, get one free' and '25% extra free' encourages overconsumption. Research also shows most people greatly under-estimate how much they eat [5].

Advice for patients to help reduce portion sizes

- Weigh food to check portion sizes until familiar with an average portion in 'the mind's eye'
- Look at portion sizes on a plate
- Use smaller plates
- Don't leave dishes on the table to encourage second helpings – plate up in the kitchen
- Tidy away leftovers before sitting down
- Look for smaller sizes of snack foods
- Women do not need the same portion sizes as men, so it is important this is reflected at mealtimes

---

Portion control is one way of ensuring that patients successfully control their energy intake. Clear guidance on portion sizes is of crucial importance (see Appendices 12, 13, 14 and Resource 26).

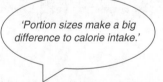

'Portion sizes make a big difference to calorie intake.'

Example of a discussion about portion control

Practitioner: '*One aspect of weight management that most people find difficult is portion sizes.*'
Patient: '*How do you mean?*'
Practitioner: '*Well, portion sizes have increased greatly over the past few decades and it means that often we end up eating more than we need.*'
Patient: '*Yes, I suppose you are right.*'
Practitioner: '*Because it is difficult, we focus quite a lot on it during our sessions.*'
Patient: '*I see.*'
Practitioner: '*I have some tips here that have been found to be helpful. Would you like to have a look and see which ones apply to you?*'
Patient: '*Sure.*'
Practitioner: '*Can I suggest you take it home and use it as a guide? Also, if you can really focus on portion sizes in your diary, keeping that helps as well.*'
Patient: '*OK.*'

Smaller portions

Beans on toast

1 slice (22 g) toast, 5 g margarine, 130 g beans = 205 kcals
2 slices (44 g) toast, 5 g margarine, 195 g beans = 356 kcals

Chilli con carne

170 g chilli, 96 g rice = 307 kcals
340 g chilli, 22 g rice = 661 kcals

Chicken curry

260 g curry, 96 g rice = 390 kcals
365 g curry, 161 g rice = 580 kcals

Lasagne

195 g lasagne = 357 kcals
430 g lasagne = 787 kcals

Macaroni and cheese

222 g macaroni and cheese = 460 kcals
385 g macaroni and cheese = 797 kcals

Pizza, thin-crust pepperoni

2 × 75 g slices = 383 kcals
4 × 75 g slices = 764 kcals
2 × 115 g slices = 586 kcals
4 × 115 g slices = 1172 kcals

Quiche lorraine

65 g quiche, 65 g coleslaw = 410 kcals
400 g quiche, 195 g coleslaw = 1980 kcals

Roast lamb

75 g = 180 kcals
125 g = 300 kcals

Shepherd's pie

240 g = 350 kcals
360 g = 526 kcals

Sausage and mash

110 g sausage, 235 g mash, 50 g gravy = 587 kcals
220 g sausage, 470 g mash, 100 g gravy = 1175 kcals

Meal ideas

Sometimes people complain of boredom when following a weight-management diet. It can be difficult when changing usual eating habits and it can help to have new ideas of suitable choices.

Breakfast ideas have already been covered. Below are some ideas for light meals and main meals.

Ideas for light meals (approx. 350 calories)

- Sandwich (2 slices bread): with different fillings, e.g. ham, cheese, tuna, salmon, egg. Add salad and low-fat spread
- Beans (120 g) on toast (2 slices)
- Cheese (50 g) on toast (2 slices)
- Salad and cold meat (2 oz) and low-fat dressing. Wholemeal roll (1 medium roll)
- Cooked pasta (3 tablespoons) salad with prawns in low-fat dressing
- Jacket potato (8 oz) and cheese (2 oz)
- Pitta bread (1) filled with cold meat (2 oz) and salad
- Ready-made sandwiches: 350 calories or less

Meal ideas for main meals (approx. 450 calories)

- Low-fat cooked mince (4 oz) with pasta (3 tablespoons), salad
- Grilled chicken portion (4 oz), vegetables and 2 egg-sized potatoes (8 oz)
- Grilled sausages (2), mashed potato (2 tablespoons) and vegetables
- Poached fish (5 oz), sweetcorn (2 tablespoons), 2 boiled potatoes (8 oz)
- Lamb casserole (4 oz), vegetable and 2 boiled potatoes (8 oz)
- Roast beef (4 oz), vegetables, 2 roast potatoes (8 oz), 1 Yorkshire Pudding
- Ready meals: 450 calories or less

Losing weight doesn't mean having to avoid dessert.

Ideas for dessert (100–150 calories)

- Yogurt (100 calories or less)
- Fruit (1–2 portions)
- Fruit in jelly
- Plain ice cream (2 scoops)
- Readymade dessert (100 calories or less)

Use minimum amounts of butter, margarine or oil.
NB Check the portion sizes.

Menu planning

Menu planning is a skill that appears to have been lost over the years. People tend to shop more frequently and buy on impulse, which may result in poor food and meal choices. Planning meals ahead of time is a vital skill for managing weight and needs to be tailored to the individual's food preferences. There is little point in giving out a set of pre-printed menus, which may not reflect relevant meals and food choices. Menu planning can be a time-consuming process and may need to be discussed over a number of visits until the patient is confident in this skill.

Using Tool 11, patients can be supported to plan breakfasts for 1 week, taking into account their current habits and preferences. The same exercise can be done for lunch and then evening meals, snacks and drinks. Once meal-planning has been completed for breakfast, encourage patients to work on another meal before the next appointment. (See Resource 23 for recipe ideas). Once patients have developed a set of menus for 1 week, they may be happy to repeat this on a weekly basis with occasional variation. Encourage patients to stick with their pre-planned menus, which can make diary-keeping an easier task.

Example of a menu-planning discussion

Patient: *'I need some ideas for what I can eat. Have you got a diet sheet?'*
Practitioner: *'I can give you some written information* [see resource list], *but when it comes to planning meals I find it helps to take into account each person's own food preference. Would you be happy to spend some time building up your own meal plans over the next few visits?'*
Patient: *'OK.'*
Practitioner: *'Which meal do you need most help with?'*
Patient: *'Evenings – I can never think what to have!'*
Practitioner: *'Let's make a list of the things you enjoy at the moment. Can we have a look at your diary to see what your favourite foods are?'*
Patient: *'OK, I just feel I need a few fresh ideas.'*
Practitioner: *'OK, let's put our heads together! There you have ideas for 1 week* [Table 8.1]. *What I'd like to suggest now is that you fill in the portion sizes* [see Appendix 12] *when you get home and then do a shopping list based on these meals. How does that sound?'*
Patient: *'Fairly straightforward.'*
Practitioner: *'See how it goes, and don't forget to continue to keep a record in your food diary. We can work on more ideas next time we meet...'*

Table 8.1   Example of 1 week's menu for evening meals

Day	Mon	Tue	Wed	Thu	Fri	Sat	Sun
Meal	Cold meat Salad Potato	Spaghetti bolognaise Salad	Fishcakes Sweet corn Boiled potato	Sausage & mash Peas	Chicken in a sauce Rice Salad	Steak Tomatoes Peas Mushroom Oven chips	Scrambled egg on toast Tomato

Although variety can be important to avoid boredom and ensure nutritional adequacy of the diet, too much variety may not be helpful either! As the variety of foods available increases, so the total amount of food consumed may increase. After meal-planning, the next step is to develop a shopping list.

Shopping

Food shopping can be very challenging for someone who is trying to control weight. Supermarkets use clever marketing strategies to encourage increased consumption and the wise food shopper has to be prepared to overcome these approaches.

Going shopping with a list, and sticking to it, is essential. Encourage patients to look at labels carefully and to compare the calorie content of different products, avoiding special offers: 'buy one, get one frees', '25% more' and so on. Buying larger amounts of food as value packs may seem like a bargain but having more available food at home is likely to lead to increased consumption. If possible, it is also a good idea to avoid shopping when hungry.

Tips for shopping wisely

- Plan ahead. Plan meals in advance and make a shopping list
- Take the shopping list and keep to it
- Avoid the tempting aisles and special offers
- Never go shopping on an empty stomach
- Don't shop on impulse
- Try shopping online to avoid temptation
- Stock up with fruit and vegetables first
- Ready meals: choose healthy options or low-calorie varieties

Encourage patients to look at labels carefully and to compare the calorie contents of different products.

Example of a discussion about shopping

Practitioner: '*I think we agreed we would talk about shopping at today's session?*'
Patient: '*Yes, and I have become very aware of how much stuff I buy that gets chucked away.*'
Practitioner: '*Maybe you can save some money as well! Can we look at when you shop and how you plan it?*'
Patient: '*Yeah. I guess I have got out of the habit of doing a shopping list.*'
Practitioner: '*It really does help if you can do a list and stick to it. Would you like to look at other things that help as well?*'
Patient: '*Sure.*'

Many local dietetic services run shopping tours, which are a very practical way of helping patients develop shopping skills.

Food labels

Food labelling can be confusing for people and it is worth spending time ensuring patients understand how to improve their understanding of food labels.

For weight management, **the calorie content is the most important figure on the label**. Encourage patients to compare the **calorie** content of foods **per serving**. This takes practice and practitioners can support patients in developing this essential skill. Encourage patients to bring in empty packets of their favourite foods and build up a supply for use as a teaching resource.

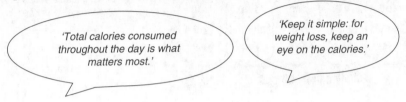

'Total calories consumed throughout the day is what matters most.'

'Keep it simple: for weight loss, keep an eye on the calories.'

Label traps

People are often misled into thinking a food is a good choice because it is labelled 'healthy', 'low-fat', 'low-carb' 'low-sugar' or 'no added sugar'. This is not necessarily the case. Sometimes, these foods contain only a few calories less, but because of the label, people tend to eat more, thinking they are eating a low-calorie food. This can result in an overconsumption of calories.

Ingredients are listed in order of weight, so the main ingredients in the packaged food always come first. That means that if the first few ingredients are high-fat ingredients, such as cream, butter or oil, the food is high in fat.

For guidance on the nutrition content of foods, some front of nutrition labels use, red, amber and green (traffic right) colour-coding, as shown in Figure 8.2 which tells you at a glance if a food has high, medium or low amounts of fat, saturated fat, sugars and salt. In short, the more green lights, the healthier the choice.

- red means high
- amber means medium
- green means low.

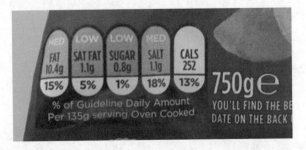

Figure 8.2   Traffic light colour coding. Courtesy of Department of Health (2011).

Some food companies use 'Guideline Daily Amounts' (GDAs) (Figure 8.3) as an alternative method of labelling. GDAs are a guide to how many calories and nutrients people can consume each day for a healthy, balanced diet. The GDA label shows the number of calories and grams of sugars, fat, saturates (saturated fat) and salt per portion of food, and expresses these quantities as a percentage of your Guideline Daily Amount.

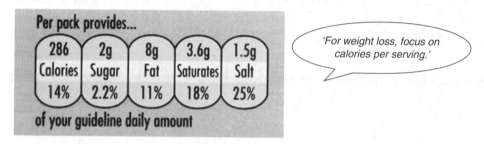

Figure 8.3   Guideline daily amounts (GDAs). Courtesy of Department of Health (2011).

For **general healthy eating,** further guidance is available on nutritional content per 100 g. The recommendation is to aim for **low amounts of fat, sugar and salt** (see Table 8.2 and Resource 24).

Table 8.2   Guidelines on the nutrient content of foods

	High	Low
Total fat	≥20 g	≤3 g
Saturated fat	≥5 g	≤1.5 g
Sugars	≥15 g	≤5 g
Salt	≥1.5 g	≤0.3 g

Guidance on reading labels

For weight loss
1 Check serving size per container.
2 Check calories per **serving**.

To ensure nutritional adequacy
3 Limit total fat, saturated fat, salt, sugar.
4 Check for adequate fibre, vitamins and minerals.

Bear in mind that some patients may struggle to read labels due to sight impairment or literacy skills.

The majority of the population consumes prepackaged foods to a greater or lesser extent and food labelling provides information on their calorie and nutrient content. However, reading labels can be difficult and practitioners have an important role in supporting patients to better understand what a label is really telling them about their food.

Cooking

Cooking healthily is an essential part of losing weight and keeping it off in the longer term. Patients should continue to cook their favourite foods but ensure the use of low-fat cooking methods.

There are plenty of good recipe books available to help inspire people with meal ideas. A list of useful books can be found in Appendix 15. Perhaps encourage patients to bring in their favourite recipes and share them with others.

Discussion about cooking

Practitioner: '*Are you keen on cooking?*'
Patient: '*Yes, everyone says I'm a good cook!*'
Practitioner: '*Great. It is worth looking at your favourite recipes to see if you can save any calories by adapting them.*'
Patient: '*If you think it will help.*'
Practitioner: '*Every little helps. Would you like some hints and tips?*'
Patient: '*Yes, please.*'
Practitioner: '*It is also really important to watch **portion sizes**.*'

Many services run 'Cook and Eat' sessions for those who need to develop their cooking skills (contact public health departments for local information).

Cooking tips

- Use low-fat cooking methods such as grilling, poaching, casseroles
- Avoid using the frying pan or use the minimum amount of oil for recipes
- Use a spray for oil and use a nonstick pan
- Trim the fat from meat and remove skin from poultry
- Use skimmed milk and cornflower for white sauces
- Use low-fat cheese in recipes
- Be careful about the amount of cheese used
- Use lean mince
- Instead of cream, try low-fat yogurt
- Use oil-free dressings

Recipe adaptation

Minced beef

Cook *lean* mince in a *dry* saucepan over a *low* heat. Stir all the time until it browns. Discard any fat (pour away, use kitchen roll to absorb or leave overnight in the fridge and remove solid fat). Add vegetables and flavourings as normal.

Calorie saving: 70 kcal per serving.

Use as a base for: spaghetti bolognese, shepherd's pie, lasagne, moussaka, chilli con carne.

White sauce

Use skimmed milk blended with cornflour rather than flour and butter/margarine.

Calorie saving: 700 kcal per pint = 70 kcal per serving.

Use for making cheese sauce, parsley sauce, onion sauce.

Cheese sauce

Make white sauce as above and add a low-fat or half-fat cheese.

Calorie saving: 72 kcal per serving

Use for lasagne, moussaka, macaroni and cheese, fish pie.

Custard

Use skimmed milk and a sweetener.

Calorie saving: 305 kcal per pint, 76 kcal per serving.

'I didn't realise I could save so many calories by making these simple changes.'

'The family are happy that I am still cooking their favourite dishes.'

Special occasions

Celebrations

Special occasions are often marked by special food. For someone trying to lose weight, this can be especially difficult. Sometimes it may be best to have a little of what is going and join in with the celebrations. Special occasions do not happen every day and will not make a big difference to overall progress if the patient gets back on track straight after the event.

Holidays

Holidays can also present a challenge. Sometimes people want to forget about their diet for 2 weeks while on holiday, but this is likely to lead to a significant weight increase, which can be very disheartening. It is better to plan ahead and adopt a 'damage-limitation' approach. It may be that the patient plans to relax a little and enjoy different foods on holiday, but in moderation and with the aim of keeping weight steady. It has been shown that people who continue to keep a food diary manage their weight much better on holiday than those who don't [6].

Discussion about holidays

Practitioner: *'Have you thought about how you are going to manage your weight on holiday?'*

Patient: *'Not really. I always put on weight when I go on holiday!'*

Practitioner: *'Maybe you can prevent that happening this time. Would you like to discuss how you might do that?'*

Patient: *'Yes, I always get depressed when it goes up.'*

Eating out

Eating out can be a big challenge. Portion sizes tend to be bigger and the range of tempting foods makes lower-calorie choices more difficult. People who successfully lose weight tend to eat mostly at home [4]. This doesn't mean eating out and weight loss are incompatible, but careful planning is required.

Tips for eating out

- If possible, decide beforehand what you are going to eat
- Three courses will take you over your calorie allowance for the day so try to stick to one or two
- Starters: choose fruit or salad. Be aware that creamy soups, rolls, butter, pâté, pastry, dressings and fried starters all add extra calories
- Main courses: choose simple dishes and go easy on sauces. Fill up with vegetables. Be aware that fried foods, added butter, oil and sauces add extra calories
- Desserts: choose ice cream or fruit
- Be careful with alcohol – drink plenty of water instead

Making healthy choices when eating out

Fast-food choices: choosing healthier options

- Burger bars: choose a burger in a bun with salad and diet drinks
  Double burgers, added cheese, mayonnaise, thick shakes, deep-fried foods
- Fish and chips: ask for a **small** portion of chips. Eat the fish and leave the batter
- Pizza: choose thin crust
  Extra toppings
- Jacket potato: choose low-calorie fillings such as baked beans, cottage cheese, tuna, chilli, vegetables
  Butter and mayonnaise
- Sandwiches: choose lean meats, fish, egg and half-fat cheese as fillings
  Add salad
  Mayonnaise and other dressings
- Steakhouses: choose grilled steak
  Larger portion size and 'extras'

Higher-calorie options

Italian

- Choose grilled meat and fish
  Sauces and butter on vegetables
- Choose tomato-based pasta dishes
  Creamy sauces and garlic bread

Higher-calorie options

Indian

- *Starters* – have a plain poppadum instead
- Choose tandoori and tikka dishes or dishes without sauces
- Choose boiled rice
- *Extras such as naan bread and side orders*

Higher-calorie options

Chinese

- Choose clear soups for starters
  All fried starters and prawn crackers
- Choose stir-fry, chow mein, chicken, prawns or beef in black bean sauce
  Sweet and sour or any other battered dishes
- Choose boiled rice

Higher-calorie options

Mexican

- Choose grilled meats or fish and salads and boiled rice
- Try burritos or fajitas but be careful with added cheese and sour cream
- Tortilla wraps without added extras
- *Extras, e.g. nachos and guacamole*

Higher-calorie options

Calorie swops when eating out

High-calorie fast food	Instead
Double cheeseburger + large fries + large Coke = 1160 kcal	Double burger + small fries + Diet Coke = 725 kcal
	Ordinary burger + small fries + Diet Coke = 485 kcal

High-calorie Italian	Instead
Garlic bread (4) = 400 kcal	Melon = 40 kcal
Spaghetti carbonara = 1070 kcal	Spaghetti arrabiata = 400 kcal
Tiramisu = 440 kcal	Ice cream = 140 kcal
Total = 1910 kcal	**Total = 580 kcal**

High-calorie Indian	Instead
Samosa = 140 kcal	Tandori chicken breast = 270 kcal
Chicken madras = 600 kcal	Boiled rice = 370 kcal
Pilau rice = 650 kcal	1 poppadum = 55 kcal
Naan bread = 280 kcal	**Total = 695 kcal**
Total = 1670 kcal	

High-calorie Chinese	Instead
Crispy seaweed = 200 kcal	
Spare ribs (4) = 560 kcal	Chicken & sweetcorn soup = 170 kcal
180 g fried rice = 625 kcal	180 g boiled rice = 370 kcal
Beef in black bean sauce = 380 kcal	Beef in black bean sauce = 380 kcal
Total = 1765 kcal	**Total = 920 kcal**

High-calorie Mexican	Instead
Tortilla chips and guacamole = 590 kcal	
Chicken fajitas = 1035 kcal	Chicken burrito = 600 kcal
Chocolate fudge cake = 400 kcal	Side salad = 150 kcal
Total = 2025 kcal	**Total = 750 kcal**

It is possible to eat out on a calorie-controlled diet, but it requires careful planning and a strong determination to stick with the plan.

Promoting physical activity

Physical activity should be promoted to improve overall health, regardless of weight.

The UK physical-activity guidelines encourage **all** adults to:

- Engage in moderate-intensity aerobic physical activity for **at least 150 minutes per week**; this activity should be spread across the week. Engaging in at least 30 minutes on 5 or more days each week is one example of how this volume can be achieved [7,8]. Alternatively, comparable benefits can be achieved through 75 minutes of vigorous-intensity activity spread across the week or a combination of moderate- and vigorous-intensity activity [8]
- Undertake physical activity to improve muscle strength on at least 2 days a week [8]
- Minimise the amount of time spent being sedentary (sitting) for extended periods [8]

Recommendations for weight management

During weight-loss phase, aim to increase to:

- **At least 45–60 minutes 5 times per week of moderate-intensity activity**   This will contribute 1800–2500 calories per week (3500 calories is approximately equivalent to 0.5 kg of body fat), emphasising the importance of combining activity with dietary changes to achieve the desired weight-loss outcome of 0.5–1 kg/week

During weight-maintenance phase, aim for:

- **At least 60–90 minutes 5 times per week of moderate-intensity activity**   A person who has lost weight is susceptible to weight regain and maintaining a high level of activity helps to sustain increased lean body mass. The impact on metabolism helps to sustain the weight lost (this would contribute 2400–3600 calories to energy expenditure, allowing for adjustment of food intake)

In practical terms: As these levels may be daunting for those who are inactive, it may be more helpful to talk to patients about becoming an 'active person', with the aim of achieving a level of activity that will help support weight maintenance. People who start from a very inactive lifestyle may take some time to reach the optimal levels of activity, so the overall health benefits need to be emphasised, along with the message that 'every calorie counts' and the importance of paying attention to both **calorie intake** and **calorie output**

As most people do not reach the minimum physical-activity requirements for overall health [10], it is challenging to help patients achieve recommendations for weight loss and maintenance. However, becoming more active is an essential strategy for successful weight management.

Practitioners can support patients in becoming more active by:

- Helping to establish current levels of activity and inactivity
- Taking any safety concerns into consideration
- Helping patients gradually build activity into everyday life, aiming to achieve the recommended levels over time
- Encouraging some structured activities, such as clubs, classes, sports, gym or organised sessions
- Encouraging activities that build muscle strength – referring on to experts, if appropriate

Listening to and actively reflecting on concerns expressed about any difficulties encountered will help engage and build motivation to become more active. Providing information in a helpful way and problem-solving in a collaborative manner are key behavioural strategies that can be used to promote physical activity.

Consider this

- Do you currently include discussions about activity in all your weight-management consultations?
- Are you doing enough to promote activity?
- What else can you do?
- What services are available in your area?

More on healthy eating

Eating a nutritionally adequate diet is essential for health. With the emphasis on calorie restriction for weight loss, it is easy to neglect this vital component of weight management. The practitioner should guide the patient towards a diet that is healthy and well-balanced. The 'eatwell plate' (Figure 8.4, Resource 25, Appendix 12) provides guidance on how to achieve this (see also Tool 12).

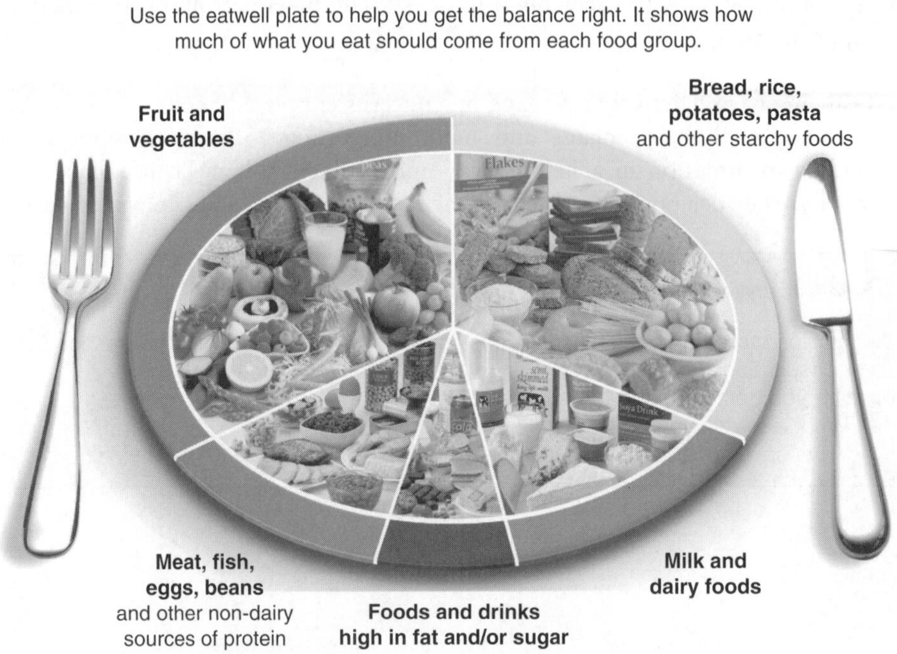

Use the eatwell plate to help you get the balance right. It shows how much of what you eat should come from each food group.

Fruit and vegetables

Bread, rice, potatoes, pasta and other starchy foods

Meat, fish, eggs, beans and other non-dairy sources of protein

Foods and drinks high in fat and/or sugar

Milk and dairy foods

Figure 8.4   The 'eatwell plate'. Courtesy of Department of Health (2011).

Guidance on portion sizes

This is an area of confusion for both practitioners and their patients. One of the differences is that **portions sizes** (on the 'eatwell plate') refer to portions from the different food groups and **serving sizes** usually refer to the amount eaten. They may or may not always be the same! For example: a 'portion' of potato is 100 g, whereas a serving may be 200 g (= 2 'portions'). *The serving on a plate may contain several 'portions'.* Table 8.3 gives guidance on portion sizes to ensure nutritional adequacy of the diet (using household measures). Table 8.4 indicates how many portions should come from each of the food groups on a 1500 and 1800 calorie diet.

Table 8.3 Household measures used for portion sizes

Food group	What counts as a portion
Bread, rice, potatoes, pasta	• 3 tbsp breakfast cereal • 1 slice bread/toast • 2–3 tbsp boiled rice/pasta • 2 egg-sized potatoes
Fruit and vegetables	• 1 medium portion vegetables • Salad • 1 medium fruit • 1 small glass fruit juice
Milk and dairy foods	• 1 glass milk (⅓ pint) • 1 pot yogurt • 1 matchbox piece of cheese (30 g)
Meat, fish, eggs, beans	• 2–3 oz cooked meat • 5 oz fish • 2 eggs • 5 tbsp baked beans
Foods containing fat	• 1 tsp butter/margarine/oil/ghee • 1 tsp mayonnaise
Extras	• Crisps, chocolate, biscuits, alcohol, etc.

Table 8.4 Recommended daily portions from each food group, equivalent to 1500 and 1800 kcal

Calories	Fruit and vegetables	Starchy foods	Dairy foods	Protein	Fats	Extras
kcals/portion	40	80	90	140	50	
1500	6 portions	6 portions	3 portions	2 portions	2	130 kcal
1800	7 portions	8 portions	3 portions	2 portions	3	180 kcal

Tool 12 can be used to help patients to check the nutritional adequacy of their diet.

Appendix 12 gives more detail on household measure that can be used with the eatwell plate.

As energy requirements increase with body weight, those with a very high BMI will be able to lose weight at intakes above 1800–2000 kcal/day.

The next step:
For those not losing weight using household measures, more precision is required with portion sizes.

Example: 1500 calories	
8:00 am	Mug of tea (350 ml) with 1/16 (35 ml) of a pint of semi-skimmed milk
8:15 am	1 wholemeal slice of bread toast (31 g), 1 teaspoon of butter (7 g) and 1 heaped tablespoon of jam (20 g) (53 kcal)
9:00 am	Mug of coffee (350 ml) with 1/16 (35 ml) of a pint of semi-skimmed milk and low-fat yogurt (150 g)
10:00 am	Mug of coffee with 1/16 (35 ml) of a pint of semi-skimmed milk
12:30 pm	2 thick-cut slices of white bread (68 g), 1 tablespoon of light mayonnaise (15 g), 1 large egg (50 g) and a smoothie (250 ml carton)
1:30 pm	1 satsuma (70 g)
3:00 pm	Mug of coffee (350 ml) with 1/16 (35 ml) of a pint of semi-skimmed milk
5:00 pm	1 apple (133 g)
7:00 pm	1 skinless chicken breast (168 g), roasted, (150 g) of a bag of frozen vegetables, boiled (63 kcal), 2 average-sized potatoes with skin (250 g), boiled
8:00 pm	2 crackers (14 g) and mature cheddar cheese (14 g) and 1 glass of red wine (190 ml)

These examples shows *exact* portion sizes for 1500 and 1800 calorie diets. This level of precision may be needed for someone who is not losing weight using household measures. Appendix 17 gives guidance on *exact* portion sizes for calorie control.

Example: 1800 calories	
8:00 am	Mug of tea (350 ml) with 1/16 (35 ml) of a pint of semi-skimmed milk
8:15 am	2 wholemeal slices of bread toast (62 g), 1 heaped teaspoon of butter (10 g) and 1 heaped tablespoon of jam (20 g)
9:00 am	Mug of coffee (350 ml) with 1/16 (35 ml) of a pint of semi-skimmed milk and a low-fat yogurt (150 g)
10:00 am	Mug of coffee with 1/16 (35 ml) of a pint of semi-skimmed milk and 1 ginger biscuit
12:30 pm	2 thick-cut slices of white bread (68 g), 1 tablespoon of light mayonnaise (15 g), 1 large egg (50 g) and a smoothie (250 ml carton)
1:30 pm	1 satsuma (70 g)
3:00 pm	Mug of coffee (350 ml) with 1/16 (35 ml) of a pint of semi-skimmed milk
5:00 pm	1 apple (133 g)
7:00 pm	1 skinless chicken breast (168 g), roasted, 180 g of a bag of frozen vegetables, boiled, 300 g boiled potatoes with skin
8:00 pm	2 rye crackers (20 g) and mature cheddar cheese (14 g), a handful of grapes (40 g) and 1 glass of red wine (190 ml)

Guidelines on healthy eating based on the 'eatwell plate'

Fruit and vegetables
How much? Aim for five or more helpings per day.
Why? Provides essential vitamins, minerals, fibre and antioxidants.

For weight loss:
- **Keep to the number and size of portions recommended**   Consuming unlimited amounts, particularly of fruits, can add significant calories to the diet
- Use low-calorie dressings
- **Hidden calories**   Added butter on vegetables and vegetables fried in batter

Bread, rice, potato, pasta and other starchy foods
How much? Aim for some starchy foods at each meal – preferably wholegrain varieties.
Why? Provides essential energy, fibre, vitamins and minerals.

For weight loss:
- **Keep to the number and size of portions recommended**   Consuming unlimited amounts of starchy foods can add significant calories to the diet
- Be careful with the amount of butter or spread used on bread and potatoes
- **Hidden calories**   Chips, fried rice and creamy sauces on pasta

Milk and dairy foods
How much? Aim for three servings per day – equivalent to 1 pint of milk.
One serving = –(200 ml) pint milk = 1 × 125 g pot of yogurt = 1 oz (25 g) cheese.
Why? They provide essential calcium for healthy teeth and prevention of osteoporosis. One in three adults develops osteoporosis, which is preventable through a healthy lifestyle. Some people are at greater risk due to hereditary or other factors, such as early menopause, hysterectomy, excessive exercising, alcohol and smoking. Adequate calcium is vital for **all** adults, along with sufficient vitamin D (from sunlight and vitamin-D-rich foods), to help with absorption.

For weight loss:
- **Keep to the number and size of portions recommended**   Consuming unlimited amounts of dairy foods can add significant calories to the diet
- Choose low-fat varieties, such as skimmed or semi-skimmed milk, low-fat or half-fat cheese and low-calorie or natural yogurts
- **Hidden calories**   Adding grated cheese to savoury dishes

Meat, fish, eggs, beans and nondairy sources of protein
How much? Aim for two or three helpings per day.
Why? They provide essential protein for the development of new cells, as well as vitamins and minerals. Choose a variety of protein sources. Red meat provides iron, which helps prevent iron-deficiency anaemia (needs to be consumed with vitamin-C-rich foods). Oily fish helps reduce the risk of death from heart disease and at least two portions of fish are recommended each week, including one portion

of oily fish (140 g). Beans and pulses (an essential source of protein for vegetarians) provide additional fibre as well as protein. Eggs are a good, cheap source of protein and iron. Limit to six per week.

For weight loss:

- **Keep to the number and size of portions recommended**   Consuming unlimited amounts of protein foods can add significant calories to the diet
- Trim fat off meat and remove skin from poultry
- Be careful with sauces and gravies
- **Hidden calories**   Fried foods – instead, grill, poach, bake or casserole

Foods and drinks high in fat and sugar
Fats:
How much? Aim for 2 teaspoons (12 g) of butter/margarine/oil per day. Replace saturated (mainly animal sources) fats with monounsaturated (olive oil and rape-seed oil) fats or polyunsaturated (vegetable oils and margarines) fats.
Why? They provide essential fatty acids as well as fat-soluble vitamins A and D.

For weight loss:

- **Keep to the number and size of portions recommended**   Consuming unlimited amounts of fatty foods can add **significant** calories to the diet. Fats are the most energy-dense foods
- Limit fried foods
- Limit foods high in fat, such as chocolate, puddings, pastry, cakes, biscuits, Danish pastries, crisps, nuts and savoury snacks
- Limit the amounts of cream, mayonnaise and high-fat dressings – use low-calorie alternatives
- **Hidden calories**   Drizzling olive oil over foods. Mayonnaise in sandwiches

Sugary foods:
How much? Aim for minimum amounts. Sugar is not an essential nutrient but there is no need to avoid it completely.
Why? It doesn't provide any nutrients other than calories.

For weight loss:

- Limit the amount of added sugar in drinks
- Limit fizzy drinks containing sugar

High-calorie fatty and sugary foods are often combined, for example puddings, cakes, biscuits and chocolate.

Drinks
For a healthy diet, adequate fluids are important and six to eight cups per day is recommended. For weight loss, low-calorie drinks should be chosen and care should be taken with alcohol, limiting intake to 2–3 units per day for women and 3–4 units per day for men.

Salt

Salt has no impact on weight but it is important to restrict its intake for the sake of overall health, in order to prevent high blood pressure, heart disease and stroke.

Any food can be consumed on a calorie-restricted diet – as long as it is counted as part of overall calorie consumption and, ideally, fits in with the 'eatwell plate' to ensure nutritional adequacy.

Becoming skilled at weight management

Becoming successful at weight management requires the development of skills as well as knowledge. Many weight-loss guidelines use very technical language to describe behavioural tools and strategies. This section aims to describe the strategies that have been shown to work in a user-friendly way. Figure 8.5 provides a sample 'Menu of Options' of key skills. The blank circles are for topics that the patient may wish to discuss (see also Tool 10).

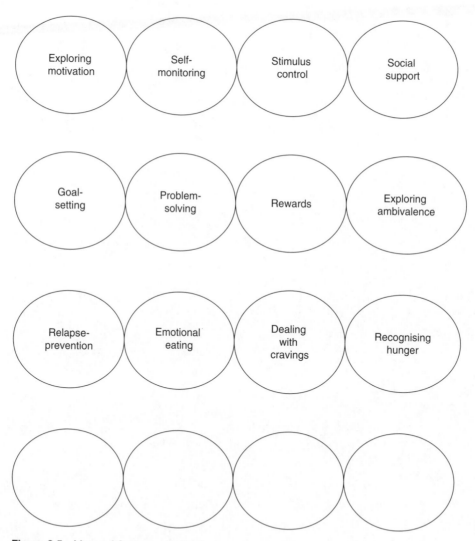

Figure 8.5   Menu of Options – key skills.

Exploring motivation ('*Do I want to, and can I?*')

The task of the practitioner is to explore, build and strengthen motivation throughout the intervention. Discussing the reasons why weight management is important and working in a supportive way helps to build confidence. Acquisition of knowledge and skills helps to further enhance confidence. Because motivation fluctuates all the time, it needs to be revisited on a regular basis. If someone is struggling and the practitioner asks, '*Does this still feel like a priority?*' it may clarify importance before moving on to explore difficulties as they occur (see Chapters 5 and 6 for more on motivation).

Self-monitoring (keeping a record)

Self-monitoring is the most valuable tool for those who are struggling with weight. It can be used to record weight, food, activity, difficult situations and so on. It also helps to record progress. It requires discipline and takes practice, but as patients build this skill they enhance their awareness of various behaviours, which leads to problem-solving. This helps build confidence, which encourages people to stay on track (Chapter 7).

> '*Learning to take a step back and look at my behaviour has helped me to become more aware.*'

Stimulus control

Many people find certain situations act as a cue or trigger for unhelpful eating and/ or activity. Temptation is part of everyday life and learning to manage these situations is important if long-term weight management is to be achieved. **Problem-solving** each situation is the best method of finding solutions. This helps people feel a greater sense of control, which in turn helps build confidence.

Example of a difficult situation (triggers or cue to unhelpful eating)

The temptation to eat crisps and nuts in the evenings: for one person, the solution may be to avoid the crisp aisle in the supermarket, but for another it may be enough to put crisps out of sight or in a harder-to-access place. Different solutions will work for different people, which is why the process of problem-solving is the best approach to use, and is most effective when used within an established collaborative helping relationship.

Problem-solving

This is an essential skill required for changing habits – replacing old eating and activity patterns with new habits. A very effective way of helping people to develop problem-solving skills in relation to weight management is to model the approach and work collaboratively with patients by going through the process (see Chapter 7 for more detail). The steps are summarised below:

Steps in problem-solving

1. Identify the problem
2. Explore the options
3. Choose preferred options
4. Develop a plan
5. Implement the plan
6. Review

---

1 **Identify the problem** People are often not fully aware of their unhelpful patterns of eating and activity. Keeping a diary (see Chapter 7) helps to highlight problem areas, which can then lead on to finding solutions. Becoming self-aware about current habits is an essential first step in the process of change.

2 **Explore the options** It is tempting for practitioners to provide lots of suggestions on what and how to change – beware! This approach can often generate resistance to change – it can feel like being told what to do, even when delivered in a 'helpful' way, such as 'How about...' or 'Do you think you could...' Instead, encourage people to think of their own alternatives before adding your own ideas. They may often look to you for guidance. When offering suggestions, always 'ask permission'. Instead of, 'Well, I think you could/should...' try, 'Would you like me to tell you what works well for others?'

3 **Choose preferred options** The chosen option must fit in with the person's everyday life. Therefore, they are the best judge of what will work for them.

4 **Develop a plan** Deciding on a plan is easy; putting it into action is the challenge. A Change Plan helps ensure that goals agreed are **Specific, Measurable, Achievable, Realistic and Time-specific.**

5 **Implement the plan** This happens outside the consultation room and it is the reason why a detailed **Change Plan** is so important in helping people convert consultation-room discussions into everyday life.

6 **Review** This vital step includes reviewing what went well/not so well, building on progress, and moving forward through Steps 1–6 once again to work through any difficulties.

Goal-setting (Developing a Plan)

Patients often struggle with planning ahead for activity, eating, social occasions and so on. Successful weight management, like any other project, requires careful planning. People are often very vague about their plans, saying, '*I'm going to cut down on food*' or '*I'm going to be more active*' – these types of vague plans are likely to end in failure. Most patients are not very skilled at setting goals for change in relation to eating and activity, so talking about 'setting goals' may not be particularly helpful. Using the everyday term of 'developing a plan' seems to make more sense to most people. A plan needs to include the **what**, the **how** and the **when** of change (see Tool 4). The more detailed the plan, the better. Encourage patients to imagine making the changes at home.

> '*Having A PLAN is the secret of success – I can't believe I never thought of it in this way before!*'

Developing a Change Plan

Successful weight management requires careful planning – the more detailed the plan, the better, and the greater the chance of success! Think about the **what**, the **how** and the **when** of your plan:

- **What** exactly are you planning to do?
  - '*I'm going to wear a pedometer and aim for 5000 steps per day.*'
  - '*I'm going to weigh my food until I get used to portion sizes.*'
  - '*I'm going to keep a careful record of my food and activity.*'
- **How** are you going to make sure it happens?
  - '*I'm going to walk round the block each morning.*'
  - '*I'm going to put the kitchen scales on the work surface.*'
  - '*I'm going to buy a special notebook and write down as I go along.*'
- **When** are you going to start?
  - '*Tomorrow!*'

Dealing with difficult situations

To further increase chances of success, people need to think about what might get in the way and how they will get round any difficulties.

Discussion about possible difficulties (barriers/obstacles)

Practitioner: 'Looking at your plan, is there anything that might get in the way or make it difficult?'
Patient: 'I guess getting up these cold mornings might be a challenge!'
Practitioner: 'What will help you get round that?'
Patient: 'If I tell my partner, he will make sure I get up.'
Practitioner: 'It sounds as if you have good support there – anything else that will help?'
Patient: 'Leaving my tracksuit and trainers ready the night before so I can just get up and go.'
Practitioner: 'What about portion sizes?'
Patient: 'I don't see any problem except dealing with leftovers.'
Practitioner: 'It is worth having a plan for how you are going to deal with that...'

Support

Research shows that people with good social support do better than those without. Part of the role of the practitioner is to offer support, but also to help patients build up their support map. Support can come from many different sources and can mean different things to different people. Types of support required may vary at different times. It is important to have a discussion about support and to include this in review appointments.

Discussion about support

Practitioner: 'You mentioned that your partner is very supportive. Have you thought about what type of support works for you?'
Patient: 'How do you mean?'
Practitioner: 'Well, some people find it helpful to be reminded about their plan if their partner sees them going off track. Others find it puts them off even more.'
Patient: 'I see what you mean!'
Practitioner: 'It is probably worth having a discussion with your partner about the kinds of things you would find helpful (and anything that is not helpful) in what he says or does. Over time, you will get to know what works best for you.'

Types of support

Encourage patients to think what kind of support works best for them, such as praise, encouragement, practical help and so on. Also, consider what doesn't work, such as comments like 'I thought you were supposed to be on a diet!' or being constantly reminded what to do.

Sources of support

There are many and varied types of support available. Be familiar with the type of support available in your local community. Again, check what suits the individual. Help people develop their own 'support map' so they do not rely totally on health-professional support. Examples:

- friends, family
- work colleagues
- group programmes, self-help groups
- the Internet, the library
- magazines/books, etc.

Enlisting support

When patients talk about getting support from family or friends, they often assume that the support will be in place just as they require it. It is important that they are specific about the type of support that they find helpful and ensure that family and friends are aware, and happy, to commit to providing this support. The more specific the request for support, the better.

Rewards

Changing established eating and activity habits is hard work. It requires commitment, focus, energy, effort and lots of practice. Using rewards as a way of reinforcing new habits is a strong component of using a behavioural approach. Patients often talk about rewards for weight loss itself, such as 'When I have lost weight, I'm going to buy new clothes'. That is a reward for the outcome, which is fine. However, to really embed new habits in order to achieve that outcome and therefore have greater chance of sustaining weight loss, the new behaviours need to be rewarded on a frequent basis.

Example of using rewards as a way of reinforcing new habits

Practitioner: 'Have you thought of how you are going to reward yourself for all this hard work?'

Patient: 'I'm going to buy new clothes when I lose the weight!'

Practitioner: 'Sounds like a good incentive. I was thinking more of all the effort you are putting in at the moment. It has been shown that people who find ways of reinforcing new habits are more likely to succeed.'

Patient: 'Give me an example...'

Practitioner: 'It can be something like treating yourself to a magazine if you have kept to your plan all week or time to do something you really enjoy, or it doesn't have to always be a 'reward'. Your partner reminding you to watch the portion sizes can be a reinforcer.'

Patient: 'I see. Something that is more likely to make it happen'

Practitioner: 'Exactly. So it shouldn't be expensive or time-consuming. It should be something you can use frequently. To add to that, talking to yourself in an encouraging way also acts as a great way of reinforcing new habits, so it's worth trying that!'

Patient: 'Mm...'

Practitioner: 'Perhaps you can start to keep a record of that in your diary as well?'

Examples of ways to reinforce new habits

- buy a magazine
- make time for a relaxing activity
- save money that would have been spent on high-calorie foods.

It is important that the person chooses what works for them, so try to avoid making suggestions that would work for you!

Exploring ambivalence (*'I want to, but I can't...'*)

Sometimes patients feel like they have hit a brick wall and need help in putting things in context. One way of doing this is to help them consider all aspects of weight management. It's called 'exploring ambivalence' but it really means looking at things from every angle. For an example, see Table 8.5.

Table 8.5   Exploring ambivalence

Advantages of making changes	Disadvantages of making changes
CHANGE • I feel better • I have more energy • My clothes fit better • My blood pressure has come down	• It is hard to avoid my favourite foods • Having to think about it all the time • Having to plan meals, shopping • Social events
Advantages of NOT making changes	**Disadvantages of NOT making changes**
No CHANGE • I could eat what I like • No planning required • Less effort • Not having to think about it	• I would probably put more weight on • My clothes would not fit • My blood pressure might go up • I would feel disappointed with myself

Using Tool 13, carefully follow the patient's statements. Looking at things impartially and totally from the patient's perspective often helps to harness and strengthen motivation. Listen out for statements like *'I've got to get back on track'*, *'I need to do it this time'*, *'I don't want to be heavier than I am now'* and reflect back to build motivation. The exercise may also highlight where some of the difficulties are, which can then lead to problem-solving.

Relapse prevention (dealing with setbacks)

Losing weight and keeping it off is an ongoing process and most people experience some slip-ups or setbacks along the way. Learning how to deal with setbacks is crucial to long-term success. First, people need to be aware that having slip-ups is a normal part of the process of learning how to manage weight effectively. How slip-ups are viewed and dealt with makes a big difference.

Sometimes patients come to a review appointment feeling very down about progress, especially if things have gone off course. The practitioner has an important role to play in helping them get back on track. Self-monitoring is an invaluable tool, along with problem-solving how to get back on track by listening empathically and reassuring the patient that setbacks happen to everyone at some point. Revisiting and exploring motivation can help rebuild commitment. Once ideas have been explored and the patient is clear about what needs to happen, encourage them to develop a Change Plan for getting back on track.

Example of a conversation about setbacks

Patient: *'I can't believe how I have slipped back – I'm just hopeless!'*
Practitioner: *'You sound very fed up. What has happened is normal for most people who try to lose weight – setbacks are bound to happen at some point. The important thing is to learn from what has happened and think how you might avoid it happening again.'*
Patient: *'So you think there is hope for me?'*
Practitioner: *'Absolutely! It would be helpful to understand what happens when you have a setback and then we can look at what you might do in the same situation on another occasion.'*

It can be helpful for the patient to rehearse what they will do if they find themselves in the middle of a setback. Different things work for different people. One example could be:

1   Say to yourself: '**Stop**' and walk away from the situation, if possible
2   Think: '**Look**' at what is happening
3   '**Listen**' to the most helpful thing you can say to yourself in the situation, e.g. *'All is not lost, tomorrow is a new day. I must stick to my plan for the rest of today'*

Emotional eating

Sometimes we eat not because we are hungry, but as a response to how we are feeling. People often use food as a comfort when they are upset or stressed. Likewise, food is often used to celebrate happy occasions. Many people eat when bored or when doing something else such as watching TV or driving.

It is important to learn to recognise what is described as 'emotional eating'. Eating for reasons other than hunger is not helpful for weight management. The first step is to recognise eating linked with emotions. Keeping a record of thoughts and feelings when eating can highlight problems in this area.

Alternatives to emotional eating

- Do something active, e.g. go for a walk
- Relaxation of any kind
- Find something that you really enjoy doing

Don't be tempted to make off-pat suggestions. This can be really difficult for someone who has used food for years to deal with emotions. Offer support, encouragement and understanding. *Overcoming Weight Problems* is a useful self-help book [11] (Resource 22). When the problem is more serious, refer for more specialist help.

Dealing with hunger

Many people mistakenly believe that they need to experience continual hunger in order to lose weight. In fact, if a person becomes too hungry they are more likely to overeat when faced with food. Learning to understand and manage hunger and urges to eat is an important part of weight management. Many people become 'out of tune' with their hunger signals. First, it is helpful to recognise the difference between physical hunger and urges to eat (cravings). Hunger is a signal caused by the body's physiological need for food. It is felt in the stomach and is often accompanied by stomach rumblings.

Using a hunger score

0   10

Not at all hungry   *Very hungry*

Ask the patient to record their hunger score at different times – before a meal, after a meal, a couple of hours after eating and so on – until they get used to recognising when they are truly hungry. It is suggested that the hunger score should be between 4 and 7 to ensure the patient does not become over-hungry or over-full.

They can be incorporated into diary-keeping.

Cravings

An urge to eat (that is not hunger) can be experienced in many different situations, such as at the sight or smell of food, when thinking about food and so on. To help people distinguish between hunger and an urge to eat, suggest that they use a scoring system to record hunger.

Dealing with cravings

Patients often say '*I have no willpower*' or '*I can't resist…*' There are many strategies that people can learn to help them overcome urges to eat (that are not hunger), and the distraction technique is one of them. The important point is that it is possible to learn ways of resisting tempting foods.

Dealing with cravings

An urge to eat that is not hunger doesn't last forever. It is like a cloud passing overhead and can be an annoyance. It usually last about 15–20 minutes. Think of something to distract you until the craving passes, such as:

● Phone a friend
● Tidy a cupboard
● Go for a walk
● Do something that requires your full attention and is not compatible with eating

---

More behavioural strategies

There are many behavioural strategies that are commonly used by people who learn to manage their eating and activity behaviours for weight management. These include:

- Do nothing else whilst eating; focus and sit down at a table
- Don't eat when watching TV or reading
- Have a glass of water with your meal
- Spend longer eating meals
- Savour your food – eat slowly and enjoy each mouthful
- Chew each mouthful thoroughly, 10–20 times
- Cut food into smaller, bite-sized pieces
- Put your knife and fork down between mouthfuls
- Use cutlery rather than fingers
- Use a smaller plate or bowl
- Put food away – out of sight
- Always shop from a list
- Never shop on an empty stomach
- Keep busy and on the move
- Break up sedentary activities like watching TV into short episodes
- Don't sit for longer than half an hour
- Plan menus for the week ahead
- Plan activity for the week ahead
- Put leftovers in the freezer
- Clean your teeth after a meal

Most of these strategies have been threaded throughout this book and integrated into the conversations. Using a behavioural approach is not about doing something to people in order to get them to change. It requires a collaborative approach using good interpersonal skills.

We have tried hard to avoid the use of jargon and to keep the approach simple, using everyday language so that the practitioner can more easily incorporate this approach into consultations.

Points to remember

- A number of strategies can be used
- The approach needs to be tailored to the individual
- The approach needs to take account of the skills of the practitioner

References

1. American Dietetic Association. Position of the American Dietetic Association: Weight Management. Journal of the American Dietetic Association 2009;109[2]:330–46.
2. Fairburn C, editor. Overcoming Binge Eating. Guilford Press; 1995.
3. Scottish Intercollegiate Guidelines Network. Management of Obesity: A National Clinical Guideline. SIGN; 2010.
4. Wyatt HR, Grunwald GK, Mosca CL, Klem ML, Wing RR, Hill JO. Long-term weight loss and breakfast in subjects in the National Weight Control Registry. Obes Res 2002 Feb;10[2]:78–82.
5. Wansink B. Mindless Eating: Why We Eat More Than We Think. New York: Bantum Dell; 2006.
6. Boutelle KN, Kirschenbaum DS, Baker RC, Mitchell ME. How can obese weight controllers minimize weight gain during the high risk holiday season? By self-monitoring very consistently. Health Psychol 1999 Jul;18[4]:364–8.
7. British Heart Foundation National Centre for Physical Activity and Health. Physical Activity Guidelines in the UK: Review and Recommendations. Loughborough University; 2010.
8. Department of Health. Start Active, Stay Active. A Report on Physical Activity for Health from the Four Home Countries' Chief Medical Officers. DoH; 2011.
9. National Institute for Clinical Excellence. Obesity: Guidance on the Prevention, Identification, Assessment and Management of Overweight and Obesity in Adults and Children. NICE; 2006.
10. The Information Centre for Health and Social Care. The Health Survey for England. NHS; 2008.
11. Gauntlett-Gilbert J, Grace C. Overcoming Weight Problems. London: Robinson; 2005.

9 Staying on Track: Weight Maintenance

> 'We can do anything we want to do if we stick to it long enough.'
>
> Helen Keller

Introduction

Traditionally, weight-management interventions focused mainly on the weight-loss phase of treatment, often discharging people from services when they had reached their target weight. It is now clear that support for weight maintenance needs to be part of treating this condition, often described as a 'chronic, relapsing disease' [1]. Practitioners, who were once satisfied if substantial weight loss could be achieved by their clients, now realise that maintaining the weight lost is of equal importance. Over the past decade, increasing efforts have been directed towards the achievement of weight maintenance. It is now known that modest weight loss (e.g. 5–10% of initial body weight) maintained for a significant amount of time can achieve positive health benefits, such as changes in blood pressure, blood glucose levels and lipid profiles [2,3].

The task of the practitioner is to help people build skills and knowledge for lifelong weight management. This needs to be highlighted at the beginning of any intervention.

Defining successful weight maintenance

A weight loss of ≥5% of initial body weight maintained for 1 year or more is the traditional definition used when evaluating the outcomes of research studies [4]. In 2001, Wing and Hill proposed defining successful long-term weight-loss maintenance as achieving an intentional weight loss of at least 10% of initial body weight and maintaining this weight for at least 1 year [5] It is estimated that over 20% of overweight and obese individuals achieve this. It appears that if weight loss is maintained for 2–5 years, the chances of longer-term success greatly increase. Stevens and colleagues recommended that long-term weight maintenance in adults be defined as a weight change of <3% of body weight [6]. In the absence of consensus, the definition below may be the most practical for everyday use:

Weight Management: A Practitioner's Guide, First Edition. Dympna Pearson and Clare Grace.
© 2012 Dympna Pearson and Clare Grace. Published 2012 by Blackwell Publishing Ltd.

Successful weight maintenance is defined as a regain of weight that is less than 6.6 pounds (3 kg) in 2 years [7].

Changes in weight

Basal metabolic weight decreases with age, and as a result, most people gain weight as they get older. This can be prevented by adjusting eating and activity levels to compensate. For those susceptible to weight gain, such as someone who has been overweight and lost weight, the risk of weight regain is high. It is challenging to push back against this natural tendency to put on weight and success in achieving weight stabilisation can be measured as a positive outcome. The majority of weight-loss interventions can realistically achieve a weight loss of 5–10% over a period of 6 months (although there will be individual variation). Patients often have difficulty in accepting these limitations of weight-loss interventions.

Causes of weight regain

There are a number of complex and varied factors involved in weight regain. These include physiological, environmental and psychological factors:

- The continued availability of tempting high-calorie foods
- The challenge of maintaining a high level of physical activity
- The decrease in metabolic rate that occurs with weight loss
- Possible hormonal adaptations to weight loss [16]

There is also the loss of one of the most powerful reinforcers present during the weight-loss phase of treatment, namely weight loss itself. Positive feedback from others often falls away after initial weight loss. All these factors can lead to feelings of frustration and discouragement, which in turn can lead to abandoning weight-control efforts [8].

The decision-making process that leads people to initiate a change in behaviour is different from those that lead to maintenance of behaviours. Decisions regarding behavioural initiation (the decision to change eating and activity habits in order to lose weight) are predicted to depend on favourable expectations regarding future outcomes (weight loss), whereas decisions regarding behavioural maintenance are predicted to depend on perceived satisfaction with received outcomes (actual amount of weight lost and its perceived benefits) [9].

What works?

Many different strategies have been evaluated, such as:

- Extended treatment
- Relapse-prevention training
- Monetary incentives

- Telephone prompts
- Peer support
- Exercise/physical activity
- Post-treatment programmes
- Continued therapist contact, when combined with behavioural therapy and relapse-prevention training
- Continued therapist contact by mail and telephone

No single strategy has been shown to be superior, but **extended support** and continued changes to **eating and activity** have been shown to be significant [10].

'The real success of a weight-management intervention is determined by how long the weight lost is maintained.'

National Weight Control Registry (NWCR) data

Data from the National Weight Control Registry (NWCR) [11] in the USA provides information on 5000 subjects who have lost weight (30 lb/13.5 kg or more) successfully and maintained that weight loss for 1 year or more.

Weight loss

- Registry members have lost an average of 66 lb (30 kg)
  - o Weight loss ranges from 30 to 300 lb (13.5–135 kg)
- They have kept it off for 5.5 years or more
  - o Ranging from 1 to 66 years!
- Some have lost weight rapidly, others very slowly

Study participants

- 80% are men and 20% are women
- The average woman is 45 years old and weighs 145 lb (65 kg)
- The average man is 49 years old and weighs 190 lb (85 kg)

Interesting facts

- 45% lost weight on their own
- 55% lost weight with the help of a weight-loss programme
- *Participants are real people living in the real world and not part of a tightly controlled research study*

Key Message: It *is* possible to lose weight and keep it off!

How did they do it?

- 98% report that they modified their food intake in some way to lose weight
- 94% increased their physical activity, most frequently by walking

There is variety in how NWCR members keep their weight off, but most report continuing with a low-calorie, low-fat diet and doing high levels of activity

Interesting facts

- 78% eat breakfast every day
- 75% weight themselves at least once a week
- 62% watch less than 10 hours of TV each week
- 90% exercise, on average, about 1 hour per day

There appears to be no single formula for success, but these findings are consistent with other studies on weight maintenance.

Implications for practice

Weight maintenance is not a static condition, where weight remains at a set point. Ideally, weight stays within a range of 2–3 kg of chosen target weight. In reality, patients often take some time to adapt to maintaining their new weight and they require skills and knowledge to enable them to do so. Throughout a lifetime, many patients will go through several periods of active weight loss followed by maintenance.

From every viewpoint, it is desirable for people who have successfully lost weight to maintain the loss and prevent weight regain. Practitioners have an important role in emphasising the chronic nature of obesity and the importance of lifelong weight management. Therefore, it is much more helpful to talk about 'weight-management programmes' which have a 'weight-loss' and a 'weight-maintenance' phase. Patients should be encouraged to make changes to diet and physical activity that they can sustain, and furthermore they should be encouraged to continue to monitor their weight and/or waist, so that awareness of any weight regain can be tracked. Patients can be encouraged to return for further support when this happens.

There clearly are implications for practitioners about how best to provide continued contact and support over an extended period of time. It may well be that support can be offered by different members of the multidisciplinary team at different times throughout the patient's life. It is also important to recognise the role that family, friends, peers and other agencies such as leisure services, commercial slimming clubs and home-based programmes can play in providing support.

Healthy habits needs to become automatic and embedded in everyday life.

Practical application

During the assessment

A comprehensive assessment of the effects of obesity on the individual's health and well being should be the starting point for any weight-management intervention. Besides assessing for risk factors linked with obesity, such as heart disease and type 2 diabetes, quality of life should also be assessed [3]. Depending on the severity of any problems highlighted, it may be more appropriate to address these concerns before or alongside weight-management treatment.

- Address realistic weight-loss expectations from the outset. Help patients decide on weight-loss targets in line with current recommendations:
  - 5% weight loss at 3 months/10% at 6 months
  - 0.5–1 kg per week/3 kg per month

Studies show that patient expectations of weight loss are usually much higher than is feasible. If weight-loss expectations are not met in terms of reaching their 'dream weight', individuals may become demoralised and abandon attempts to maintain their weight. Emphasising the health benefits of modest weight loss can be helpful in these circumstances.

Discuss the need for lifelong weight management – not just initial weight loss.

During the weight-loss phase

- Encourage patients to make a good start. Initial weight loss has been shown to be a predictor of weight-loss maintenance [12]. So, starting a weight-management programme when the timing is right and when the person can focus on making changes to eating and activity habits is crucial
- Encourage changes to eating and activity habits that are sustainable long-term
- Encourage healthy food choices, regular eating patterns – including breakfast – and reduced frequency of snacks
- Encourage self-monitoring to help build self-awareness and the ability to develop coping strategies, including dealing with hunger, cravings, social situations and holidays
- Encourage flexible restraint rather than strict dieting rules. This includes the ability to compensate for a higher-calorie meal with a lower calorie intake the next day or the ability to bank calories if going out for a special occasion
- Encourage decreasing sedentary behaviours and increasing activities that can be built into everyday life

- Encourage viewing some setbacks as normal and developing ways of coping with these setbacks in a balanced fashion (using problem-solving skills)
- Encourage patients to care for themselves and to find ways of encouraging themselves in the effort they are making
- Encourage patients to set realistic goals and to take a stepwise approach. Be generous with your affirmations and encouragement
- Encourage patients to build a network of support

The task of the practitioner is to help patients develop the knowledge and skills required to lose weight successfully and keep it off long-term. Ultimately, patients should become their own best 'resource' but they may still need ongoing help and support at different stages to ensure continued success.

During the weight-maintenance phase

Maintenance of weight lost may be the greatest challenge facing overweight people. Evolving practice continues to test different approaches in line with current evidence. Many services offer continued contact through the use of drop-in sessions. Telephone, email, text messages and social networking are also increasingly being used. Some services offer more formal structured sessions at set points post-treatment.

What is clear is that services need to develop models of continuous care which will ensure that patients are adequately supported to prevent weight regain. Until research findings are clear, different approaches will need to be tried and evaluated. It may be that the maintenance phase needs to be tailored to each individual within the limits of available resources.

Physical activity

Research has highlighted the importance of physical activity, along with establishing healthy eating habits, in helping prevent weight regain. Because of this, working towards recommended levels of activity needs to be part of a weight-management intervention from the start. Individuals will vary in their initial levels of fitness and building activity needs to be encouraged throughout the programme. At the end of the weight-loss phase, many services refer patients on to local physical-activity experts for an assessment (if this has not already taken place). They can then be encouraged to join local schemes such as walking clubs or other leisure service facilities. This helps to keep patients engaged with services for extended periods, fulfilling the recommendations from current research findings.

Physical-activity recommendations for healthy adults aged 18–65 years
Current public-health recommendations for physical activity are for **at least 150 minutes of moderate-intensity activity each week**, which provides substantial benefits across a broad range of health outcomes for sedentary adults [13,14].

This dose of exercise may be insufficient to prevent weight gain in some people, and they may require additional exercise or caloric restriction to minimise the likelihood of further weight gain.

Physical activity recommendations for weight maintenance

Aim for 60–90 minutes per day of moderate-intensity activity [2,3].

In addition to aerobic exercise, people should engage in resistance training and flexibility exercises at least twice a week. This will promote the maintenance of lean body mass, improve muscular strength and endurance, and help preserve function, all of which enable long-term participation in regular physical activity and promote quality of life.

Muscle-strengthening activity

To promote and maintain good health and physical independence, adults will benefit from performing activities that maintain, or increase, muscular strength and endurance for a minimum of 2 days each week, using the major muscle groups (legs, hips, back, abdomen, chest, shoulders and arms). Muscle-strengthening activities include:

- Stair-climbing
- Lifting weights
- Working with resistance bands
- Doing exercises that use your body weight for resistance (e.g. push ups, sit ups)
- Heavy gardening (e.g. digging, shovelling)
- Yoga and similar resistance exercises that use the major muscle groups

NB Ensure all safety considerations are met before recommending exercise

Healthy eating habits

These need to be maintained throughout life to prevent weight regain and in order to contribute to optimum health. Regular eating habits, portion control and food intake based on the 'eatwell plate' should be encouraged.

Monitoring weight changes

This is a crucial aspect of weight maintenance. If people are not monitoring what is happening to their weight, they will not be aware when and if weight starts to increase. Recent research suggests daily weighing [15] may be helpful.

Regular weight and/or waist checks are important and need to be part of the weight-maintenance plan. Agreeing a weight range to be maintained is recommended – that is, an upper and lower limit. Usually the range is 3–4 kg. People need to be aware of weight changes when they happen and be able to respond appropriately. It is helpful to analyse the reason for weight gain and to take steps to create a calorie deficit through changes to eating and activity. Self-monitoring helps to refocus. Many people learn to manage their weight by adjusting their food intake and activity over a period of time, although in reality, weight maintenance often consists of short bouts of weight loss with subsequent readjustment as weight gain occurs. This is followed by a period of weight stabilisation. It appears that if people manage to successfully maintain their weight for a period of 2 years, they are more likely to maintain lifelong [5].

Learning how to deal with setbacks

It is important that patients are prepared for setbacks during the weight-maintenance phase and that they are equipped with the knowledge and skills to deal with setbacks effectively, rather than seeing every setback as a catastrophe and giving up all efforts (see more on dealing with setbacks in Chapter 8). Having easily accessible support is important and services need to recognise the importance of being able to offer support when required.

Particular difficulties that may need more expert help include:

- weight cycling
- dissatisfaction with body image
- binge eating
- anxiety/depression.

These should have been addressed at the outset of treatment, but sometimes difficulties only emerge at a later stage and need to be dealt with regardless of the patient's weight.

Conclusion

Undoubtedly, there are enormous benefits to be gained from weight management for the patient, the practitioner, the NHS and the economy as a whole. Many practitioners describe a high degree of job satisfaction when they can not only see the clinical benefits but when patients report significant improvements in their overall quality of life, energy levels, mobility, mood, self-confidence and physical health, which literally 'add years to life and life to years'.

The challenge is to convince health care providers, overweight people and the general public that obesity is a complex, chronic condition that can only be managed effectively through lifelong care.

Consider this

When your patients reach their agreed target weight, what steps do you take to support weight maintenance?

- Refer to a weight-maintenance programme?
- Ensure they have a **plan** for weight maintenance?
- Discuss maintaining healthy eating habits?
- Discuss the importance of increased levels of physical activity, including muscle-strengthening exercises?
- Ensure plans are in place for continued support?

References

1. Bray GA. Obesity is a chronic, relapsing neurochemical disease. Int J Obes Relat Metab Disord 2004 Jan;28[1]:34–8.
2. National Institute for Health and Clinical Excellence. Obesity: Guidance on the Prevention, Identification, Assessment and Management of Overweight and Obesity in Adults and Children; 2006.
3. Scottish Intercollegiate Guidelines Network. Management of Obesity: A National Clinical Guideline. SIGN; 2010.
4. Institute of Medicine. Weighing the Options: Criteria for Evaluating Weight Management Programs. Washington, DC: National Academy Press; 1995
5. Wing RR, Hill JO. Successful weight loss maintenance. Annu Rev Nutr 2001;21: 323–41.
6. Stevens J, Truesdale KP, McClain JE, Cai J. The definition of weight maintenance. Int J Obes (Lond) 2006 Mar;30[3]:391–9.
7. National Heart Lung and Blood Institute Obesity Education Initiative. Expert Panel of the Identification, Evaluation, and Treatment of Overweight and Obesity in Adults; 2000.
8. National Obesity Forum. Long Term Maintenance; 2006.
9. Rothman AJ. Toward a theory-based analysis of behavioral maintenance. Health Psychol 2000 Jan;19[1 Suppl.]:64–9.
10. Perri M, Corsica JA. Improving the Maintenance of Weight Lost in Behavioural Treatment of Obesity. Handbook of Obesity Treatment. New York: Guilford Press; 2002.
11. Klem ML, Wing RR, McGuire MT, Seagle HM, Hill JO. A descriptive study of individuals successful at long-term maintenance of substantial weight loss. Am J Clin Nutr 1997 Aug;66[2]:239–46.
12. Elfhag K, Rossner S. Who succeeds in maintaining weight loss? A conceptual review of factors associated with weight loss maintenance and weight regain. Obes Rev 2005 Feb;6[1]:67–85.
13. British Heart Foundation. Physical Activity Guidelines in the UK: Review and Recommendations. BHF National Centre for Physical Activity and Health, Loughborough University; 2010.

14. Department of Health. Start Active, Stay Active. A Report on Physical Activity for Health from the Four Home Countries' Chief Medical Officers. DoH; 2011.
15. Wing RR, Tate DF, Gorin AA, Raynor HA, Fava JL, Machan J. STOP regain: are there negative effects of daily weighing? J Consult Clin Psychol 2007 Aug;75[4]:652–6.
16. Sumithran MB, Prendergast LA, Delbridge E, Purcell K, Shulkes A, Kriketos A, Proietto J. Long-term persistence of hormonal adaptations to weight loss. N England Journal of Medicine 2011;17:365.

10 Getting the Most out of Brief Contacts

'Nothing is a waste of time if you use the experience wisely.'

Rodin

Introduction

Successful weight management is associated with more frequent and/or longer contact sessions. It is recommended that interventions allow sufficient time for consultations – plan to provide repeat consultations and arrange frequent follow-up appointments over a period of 3–6 months [1]. The focus of this book is on one-to-one interventions where sufficient time is allocated for a thorough assessment and to develop tailored plans that meet the weight-loss and -maintenance needs of the individual.

However, given the increasing numbers of obese patients, treatment demand often overwhelms current service provision. Whilst it is important to consider the most effective use of limited time and resources, it is equally important to acknowledge the need to develop high-quality services that have sufficient resources to meet current treatment recommendations, thereby maximising outcomes achieved and improving the patient's experience of treatment.

What is a brief contact?

This chapter explores when and where brief weight-management contacts are likely to occur and what might be a productive use of those conversations, from both the patient and the practitioner's perspectives. A brief contact can be:

1   A single encounter
2   A number of brief consultations (brief interventions)

Weight Management: A Practitioner's Guide, First Edition. Dympna Pearson and Clare Grace.
© 2012 Dympna Pearson and Clare Grace. Published 2012 by Blackwell Publishing Ltd.

A brief contact (single encounter)

A brief contact describes a short intervention 'one-off', delivered opportunistically and taking 3–5 minutes (though it can be longer). It can be stand alone or as part of a longer conversation about health and/or lifestyle factors which influence health. A brief contact usually involves initiating a conversation and engaging the person in further discussion about weight. Is it a concern and do they feel able to undertake changes to their eating and activity at this point in time?

If the patient is interested, the practitioner can help them decide on the best way forward and signpost towards the most appropriate service (which could include allocating time for a longer conversation with the practitioner).

It is not about giving advice for weight management as this very much depends on the individual's starting point, which requires a proper assessment. Giving blanket advice or lots of hints and tips may be counterproductive. The conversation can be backed up by the use of a good information leaflet (Resources 7, 9 or 27).

Limitations of brief contacts

Obesity is a chronic condition and its management often demands ongoing care, which can present numerous opportunities to intervene. However, it is important to recognise the limitations of brief contacts as opposed to more structured intensive programmes. Changing eating and activity behaviours is complex and simple BMI checks with advice to 'eat less and exercise more' or the provision of lots of helpful suggestions are unlikely to be effective for many people.

Brief interventions

'Brief intervention' is a generic term referring to a variety of encounters with a patient that require relatively little time. Brief interventions emerged from addictions treatment research, which found that interventions for alcohol problems consisting of one to three sessions of approximately 5–30 minutes were as effective as more intensive interventions and more effective than no intervention.

The National Obesity Observatory has described brief interventions (for weight management) as ranging from a single session providing information and advice to a number of sessions of motivational interviewing or behaviour-change counselling [2].

Brief interventions have been shown to be effective in addictive behaviours [2], but it is unclear whether this translates to weight management and there is a need for more research to explore the potential for this approach.

Getting the most out of brief contacts

The first step towards change is engagement, and brief contacts are an opportunity to initiate discussion about weight, influence motivation and signpost appropriate interventions. It is important that this is done well in order to optimise effectiveness.

Unhelpful approaches

Given the influence of weight on many aspects of health, practitioners are encouraged to discuss excess weight with overweight and obese individuals when the opportunity arises [3]. It is tempting to use every contact as an opportunity to try to persuade the patient to lose weight. However, persuasion linked with advice-giving has been shown to reduce patient autonomy and increase resistance to change [4]. It is important that raising the issue of overweight is done at the right time and in a skilful way. Talking about weight with an overweight or obese patient can be a sensitive subject and if done badly can damage the helping relationship and the patient's self-esteem and/or prevent them from seeking support from health care altogether [5].

'The person should not leave the consultation feeling worse about themselves.' [6]

'"First, do no harm" applies in this area of health just the same as any other.'

When considering how to maximise the benefits from brief contacts for weight management, it may be helpful to consider these contacts from the patient's perspective. Managing weight is a different experience for each individual. Some people maintain a healthy weight without any conscious effort; others maintain a healthy weight by being mindful of what they eat and their levels of activity. Those who gain weight fall into many categories, such as those who gain weight after a life event, including a change in job, marital status, pregnancy or smoking cessation. Others may have struggled with their weight all their lives and tried many different approaches. The first step for the practitioner is to gain an understanding of the patient's perspective about their weight.

If at any point the patient becomes defensive or disinterested, it is a signal to the practitioner that the conversation is not going well – for example if the patient says, *'Look, I have been told this many times before – I'm sick of everyone telling me to*

Useful steps when time is limited

1 Raise the issue in a sensitive way
2 Engage in a helpful conversation about weight – explore motivation

Then, if the client is interested/engaged:

3 Discuss options, providing information in a helpful way
4 Signpost an appropriate intervention best suited to meet their individual needs
5 Offer support

lose weight!' or looks uncomfortable and stops engaging in conversation. Don't plough on with your own agenda and ignore the situation or try to persuade, frighten or cajole the patient into doing something about their weight. Consider what might be happening: the patient may be embarrassed about their weight or they may simply have other priorities. Reflect on your consulting style and ensure reflective listening skills are being used to build rapport. It may also be helpful to periodically step back and consider your own attitudes to obesity and how these can influence the helping relationship (see Chapter 2 for more on attitudes).

> *'The helping relationship is of prime importance when setting the scene for changing behavior.'* [7,8]

Raising the issue

Discussing weight can be a sensitive topic for both patients and practitioners, so it is important that it is raised in a skilful way in order to enhance the helping relationship. Context and timing make a difference. If someone attends for a health care appointment about a concern unrelated to weight, they may not appreciate the issue of weight being included in the conversation. Opportunistic weight screening is now encouraged [3], so it is essential to ensure that the effectiveness of that contact is optimised.

What is likely to be unhelpful

'You need to do something about your weight' or *'You wouldn't have these health problems if you lost weight.'*

Patients may feel more defensive if they believe they are being told off or their self-worth may decline further if they feel they are being blamed for their situation. This is not a good starting point for engaging their interest.

What is likely to be more helpful

It may be appropriate to say, *'My computer tells me that you have not had an overall health check recently. Do you mind if I check your weight and blood pressure while you are here?'*

If weight is related to the presenting condition, the practitioner might say, *'I wonder if you are aware that if you lost some weight, it could help your —?'* [See more on raising the issue in Chapter 5, page 60.]

Engaging in a helpful conversation and exploring motivation

In order to initiate weight management, people need to be engaged in the process; they need to be motivated. Practitioners are in a powerful position to influence motivation by raising the issue in a sensitive way and exploring what weight means for the individual patient. Is it something that is important to them, and if so, do they feel able to undertake changes to eating and activity at this point in time?

What is likely to be unhelpful

Telling the patient what to do: *'Now hop on the scales!'* or *'You need to eat less...'*
Judgemental comments: *'Oh dear, your weight has gone up again!'*
Labelling: *'You are obese!'*
Telling the patient why it is important: *'You really ought to lose weight because...'*
Being overoptimistic: *'Of course you can do it!'*
Dismissing concerns: *'Never mind, we will soon get you losing weight!'*

What is likely to be more helpful

Inviting the patient to be weighed: *'Would you like to step on to the scales?'*
Giving feedback in a neutral way and inviting a response: *'Your weight today is —. Is that what you expected?'*
Offering information: *'Would you like to know where it fits on the charts?'* If yes: *'Your weight is above in the normal range for your height.'*
Exploring importance: *'Is losing weight a priority for you at the moment?'* If yes, explore their reasons – this helps build and strengthen motivation. If no, acknowledge, accept (don't try to persuade!) and offer to revisit at another time.
Exploring confidence: *'Do you feel able to consider changes to your eating and activity in order to lose weight at the moment?'*
Acknowledging any perceived difficulties: *'You are concerned that you may not be successful because you have tried many times without success?'*
Offering support: *'Would it be helpful if we consider what options are available to you and what support I can offer?'*

Is now the right time?

Discussions about weight need to consider the issue in relation to the rest of the patient's life, their overall health and other commitments that may affect their decision to begin a weight-management plan. In some instances it may be better to wait until the patient can prioritise managing their weight and give full commitment to the time and effort required to instigate and sustain changes to eating and activity behaviours. It is helpful in such situations to show a willingness to revisit at a later stage: *'Perhaps we can revisit this at another time when things are more settled for you?'*

Discussing options

Provide information on the options available and involve the patient in choosing the option which they believe will meet their needs. The practitioner has a role in guiding the patient towards the option(s) that is/are likely to be most suitable for them. This should link with local care pathways.

Examples:

- Some people may prefer to manage their own weight
- Others may prefer to manage their own weight but attend for regular review
- Some people may prefer to attend a slimming referral scheme
- Others may wish to been seen for one-to-one support
- Others may need specific help with management of co-morbidities
- Some may need to combine a therapeutic diet with weight management, e.g. coeliac disease, and require a referral to a dietician for specialist advice
- Those with higher BMIs and existing co-morbidities may need referral to a specialist obesity service
- Medication may need to be considered for those who have already tried lifestyle approaches (depending on BMI)
- Bariatric surgery may be need to be considered for those with higher BMIs where weight is adversely impacting on their health or quality of life and comprehensive lifestyle programmes have not been effective [3] – see local pathways
- Other problems may be highlighted which require referral to appropriate services

What is likely to be unhelpful

Responding without listening and checking that you have understood, for example:

- *'Oh no, you don't want to do that!'*
- *'You can't have the tablets until I see that you are motivated.'*
- *'You have to show you can lose weight before I will refer you.'*
- *'That's a load of rubbish! There is only one way to lose weight – eat less and exercise more. It's quite straightforward.'*

What is likely to be more helpful

Listening carefully, acknowledging what the client says and providing information in a helpful way by:

Checking: *'You would like to attend a slimming club/exercise class/medication/surgery.'*
Asking: *'Shall we discuss that option?'*
Providing information that is relevant for that person:

- *'We operate a "slimming-on-referral" scheme. I can provide you with some details…'*
- *'The programme that I run for individuals involves attending x number of times for x weeks and then reviewing progress. Each appointment last for –. Before enrolling on the programme, I arrange an initial visit to go through things together and get a full understanding so we can work out what works best for you…'*
- *'Surgery might be the best option for you, but it is only considered when all other options have been tried. Can we discuss what you have already tried?'*

Checking: *'What do you make of that?'*
(See more about providing information in a helpful way in Chapter 7, page)

Some patients may want to pursue unsuitable options:

- Medication without a comprehensive lifestyle programme in place
- Bariatric surgery when they have not tried a comprehensive lifestyle programme
- A non-evidence-based approach

Signposting the most suitable option

Taking into account local pathways and available resources, discuss the options available with the patient and agree a way forward, signposting the most suitable option for that individual.

What is likely to be unhelpful

Being overoptimistic:

- *'That's the answer for you!'*

Warning:

- *'Remember how ill your dad was before he died. If you don't do something about your weight, you will end up in the same situation!'*

What is likely to be more helpful

Making the referral:

- *'Now that you are keen to pursue this option, I can arrange that for you. Would you like me to give you any more details about this option? I will write a letter and you will receive an appointment... I hope you find it helpful.'*

If you are going to see the person again for another reason, continue to express interest:

- *'I will be interested to hear how you get on.'*
- *'How are things going with your weight-management plan?'*

Continuing to offer support

For patients, weight management is lifelong and there is a role for ongoing support. It may be that when a particular treatment option is chosen, the patient is referred on and attends the service for 6 months or more. However, plans need to be developed to determine what happens subsequently. In some instances, patients may feel their weight is well controlled after treatment and there is no need for ongoing support, although they are at risk of weight regain over time. Supporting patients in tracking their weight lifelong is an important part of sustained weight management.

If someone attends a programme and fails to lose weight, it is essential to recognise and respect the effort made, leave the door open for future discussions on weight management and continue to optimise the care provided for any obesity-associated co-morbidities.

Brief interventions (if ongoing support includes brief review appointments)

What *not* to do

- Offer vague 'eat less and exercise more' advice:
  - *You need to lose weight. Just cut down on the fats – crisps, biscuits, that kind of thing – and eat more fruit and veg.'*
  - *'Make sure you do plenty of exercise.'*
- Try to give as much advice as possible during consultations:
  - Better to give one or two pieces of advice that are **specific** and **tailored** for the patient to follow
- Offer advice and leave for a long period:
  - Try to see them again within 2–4 weeks
- Give lots of different leaflets:
  - Better to give one leaflet that the patient is likely to read
- Keep seeing the patient for weight management, if progress is not being made

Making the best use of available time for ongoing brief contacts

- Have a protocol   Agree a clear plan of what is going to be covered during the brief contacts – e.g. weight checks only or weight checks with brief advice – and how often, etc
- Use good-quality information leaflets and booklets (e.g. Resources 7, 9 and 27) Ensure that these resources have been approved and agreed locally
- Recognise the limitations of brief contacts for weight management   They may be an effective strategy for some patients but not for others. If progress is not being made, review and agree a way forward, e.g. referral to a more intensive programme or discharge from weight-management intervention if it is not working

Implications for services

- Evaluation of existing services (see Chapter 11)   Like all other services, the effectiveness of brief contacts needs to be evaluated:
  - Are they working?
  - Are there improvements that could or need to be made?
  - Safety: is there any potential for harm?

- **Protocols:**
  - o   Practitioners: have a clear plan of who does what (clarification of roles and responsibilities)
  - o   Patients: have a clear plan of action for each individual
- **Training needs**   Consider what skills and knowledge are required for brief contacts:
  - o   Don't assume 'every practitioner can do weight management'
  - o   Ensure that practitioners have the right knowledge and skills for their role
- **Ongoing continuing professional development:**
  - o   Ensure all practitioners are up to date with evidence-based practice
  - o   Build in clinical supervision

Examples of brief contacts

- A district nurse sees a patient at home after surgery. The patient is likely to be immobile for several months. This may be an ideal opportunity to discuss with the patient how easy it is to put weight on when immobile (especially if food consumption is not reduced to compensate for reduced energy expenditure)
- A health visitor visits a new mother at home. The mother is/is not be overweight herself. She has another toddler whom she describes as 'chubby'. This may be an ideal time to discuss family eating and activity
- A practice nurse sees a young woman who is thinking of coming off the pill with a view to getting pregnant. The patient has a BMI of 27. The importance of being a healthy weight pre- and during pregnancy should be discussed
- A GP or nurse sees a patient who has weight-related health problems
- A routine health screen
- A cardiac rehabilitation nurse sees someone who has just had a cardiac event
- A physiotherapist sees someone whose weight is contributing to their condition
- An occupational therapist sees someone whose mobility is being hampered by their weight
- A community health worker works with families in which one or more members are overweight
- A leisure service officer sees someone who would benefit from weight-management advice

The temptation is to highlight the weight problem and give brief advice and lots of encouragement. Think carefully about what is going to be the most effective use of the time you have together; sometimes less is more. If the patient goes away thinking seriously about weight loss and determined to do something about it, that is a better result than their feeling totally overwhelmed. If the patient has the opportunity to discuss what their weight means to them – perhaps explain why they find it so difficult – they are more likely to feel understood and are more likely to engage in the conversation and explore options for change.

What is likely to be unhelpful

Practitioner: '*You need to do something about your weight!*'
Patient: '*I know... but...*'
Practitioner: '*Well, cutting down on the fats is a good place to start – crisps, biscuits, chocolate and that kind of thing.*'
Patient: '*But I don't eat that much.*'
Practitioner: '*Well, I'm sure you can find room to cut down. And don't forget to exercise!*'

At the end of the consultation, the patient leaves feeling annoyed and not understood.

What is likely to be more helpful

This conversation takes the same amount of time as the example above.

Practitioner: '*Are you happy to discuss how losing weight would help your — ?*'
Patient: '*OK, but I have tried and nothing seems to work!*'
Practitioner: '*You sound disheartened with your previous attempts.*'
Patient: '*Yes, and now my job is so stressful that I can't get to the gym anymore.*'
Practitioner: '*That makes it more difficult.*'
Patient: '*Yes, and the job means eating away from home a lot more as well.*'

If we do nothing else, make sure patients feel respected and understood.

Consider this

- How do I manage brief weight-management contacts at the moment?
- Do I have a clear protocol?
- Do I have the appropriate knowledge?
- Do I have the skills required?
- When did I last have an update?
- Do I have clinical supervision for this aspect of my job?
- How do I measure the effectiveness of a brief contact?

Conclusion

There is much to be gained from making the most of brief contacts and using these interventions effectively in reducing the burden of obesity. However, careful consideration needs to be given to how to optimise these opportunities.

References

1. National Institute for Clinical Excellence. Obesity: Guidance on the Prevention, Identification, Assessment and Management of Overweight and Obesity in Adults and Children. NICE; 2006.
2. Cavill N, Hillsdon M, Anstiss T. Brief Interventions for Weight Management. Oxford: National Obesity Observatory; 2011.

3. Department of Health. Healthy Weight, Healthy Lives: A Toolkit for Developing Local Strategies. http://www.dh.gov.uk/en/Publicationsandstatistics/Publications/DH_088968; 2008.
4. Rollnick S, Mason P, Butler C. Health Behavior Change: A Guide for Practitioners. Churchill Livingstone; 1999.
5. Foster G. Goals and strategies to improve behavior-change effectiveness. In Bessesen DH, Kushner R. Evaluation and Management of Obesity. Hanley & Belfus; 2002.
6. Miller, B. Cardiff: Motivational Interviewing Workshop; 2011.
7. Brownell KD, Cohen LR. Adherence to dietary regimens 1: an overview of research. Behavioral Medicine 1995;20:149–54.
8. Brownell KD, Cohen LR. Adherence to dietary regimens 2: components of effective interventions. Behavioral Medicine 1995;20:155–64.

11 Evaluating Individual Weight-management Interventions

'If you do what you've always done, you'll get what you always got.'

Mark Twain

Introduction

- How do we know whether our weight-management activities make a difference?
- Are treatment goals being achieved?
- Are users satisfied with their experience?
- Are users satisfied with the outcomes achieved?
- How could we improve interventions and services in the future?

The only way to identify whether, and to what extent, we make a difference is to monitor and evaluate the care we provide. Although evaluation requires additional time, it is an excellent investment towards the delivery of high-quality weight management care. Given current funding pressures, there is a need to demonstrate efficiency and effectiveness and provide '**more with the same not more of the same**' [1]. Alongside this is the increased focus in the NHS on developing services responsive to patients' needs and which involve users in the development of care. Scrutinising the **quality** of weight management interventions in terms of their effectiveness, patient experience and safety should be prioritised.

Quality assurance has been defined as 'assuring a specified degree of excellence through continuous measurement and evaluation' [2]. In practice this means having systems set up locally which address clinical and self-governance. This may include activities such as clinical audit, setting and monitoring standards, risk management, health and safety, evidence-based practice, benchmarking, involving users in the development of services and education and training.

Weight Management: A Practitioner's Guide, First Edition. Dympna Pearson and Clare Grace.
© 2012 Dympna Pearson and Clare Grace. Published 2012 by Blackwell Publishing Ltd.

What is monitoring and evaluation?

Some definitions

Monitoring

This is the *routine* tracking of key aspects of the weight-management programme. For example, the number of people attending their first appointment.

Evaluation

This is the *episodic* assessment of collected information so a judgment can be made about whether, and to what extent, the 'activity' has achieved what it set out to do. For example, *to what extent did the clinical outcomes at week 24 of the weight-management programme meet the goals identified at the start?*

An outcome

This is the impact of the weight-management activity, such as $x\%$ of patients stopped gaining weight or $x\%$ of patients lost 0–3% weight.

An output

This describes the processes linked with the weight-management activity, such as:

• How many people opted into the service and booked an appointment?
• How many people completed the programme?
• How many patients permitted their weight to be measured?

The seven pillars

Quality can be described according to the seven pillars of clinical governance. It is beyond the capacity of this book to describe these in great detail, but further guidance can be obtained from 'Understanding Clinical Governance and Quality Assurance: Making it Happen' [3].

1) Clinical effectiveness

'Do the right thing to the right person at the right time in the right place.'

In practice:

• Implement the NICE and SIGN national obesity guidelines
• Develop local protocols and guidelines

2) Audit

This can be retrospective or concurrent and is the means of monitoring clinical practice and highlighting where problems may exist so they can be addressed. Results are usually measured against a standard such as NICE recommendations.

3) Risk management

This requires systems to be developed to identify risks to patients and staff and reduce the chance of mistakes occurring in the future.

In practice, consider:

- Complying with weight-management protocols
- Learning from mistakes
- Risk assessment of furniture for the obese patient

4) Education and training

Ensuring staff develop and maintain the skills and competencies necessary to deliver high-quality weight-management care is critical. There is a commonly held notion that weight management requires few specialist skills and can be delivered by staff with limited training in nutrition, physical activity and/or behavioural approaches. Given the complex causes of obesity and the well-recognised challenge of managing this chronic and relapsing condition, optimal education and training in obesity is essential [4].

In practice, consider:

- Self-reflecting on current skills and competencies
- Ensuring current knowledge is evidence-based and up to date
- Attending interpersonal skills/behaviour-change training courses
- Joining local obesity interest groups (local Association for the Study of Obesity meetings, National Obesity Forum conferences, Dietitians in Obesity Management group (DOM UK) (see Part 4 for contact details))
- Shadowing specialists
- Undertaking specialist training

5) Patient and public involvement

Gathering patient feedback is important if practice is to be improved and services are to meet patient needs.

In practice, consider:

- Patient feedback questionnaire (see section on patient-reported experience measures (PREMs) later in this chapter)
- Involving patients in the design of programmes, which could be in the form of focus groups

6) Using information and IT

This is about ensuring that systems are in place which collect information appropriately and use it to improve the quality of patient care.

7) *Staffing and staff management*

A well-motivated and well-managed team is more likely to deliver high-quality consistent care. Supporting staff to develop the skills and competencies necessary is an integral aspect of developing a team to feel confident in their ability to make a difference. Ensuring clinical supervision is in place is part of this process.

Evaluation can mean different things to different people

Different groups will have different ideas about what is important to include in evaluation.

For example, a service user may be interested in:

- *Am I achieving what I want to achieve?'*
- *'Does the experience of this treatment meet my needs and expectations?'*
- *'Is this service easily accessible?'*

Practitioners on the other hand may want to know:

- *'Does my advice and support help patients improve their eating and activity behaviour?'*
- *'Does my advice and support help patients lose meaningful amounts of weight?'*
- *'Do I have the skills and competencies required to deliver a high-quality intervention?'*

This highlights the importance of including all interested parties in the planning stages to ensure all views are considered. For outcomes to be meaningful to patients, it is important to involve users in their development – user-developed outcomes are called PROMs (Patient-Reported Outcome Measures). Changes in symptoms associated with their weight (e.g. shortness of breath, back pain, fatigue), changes in how they function (e.g. can they get washed and dressed, are they socially isolated) or other quality-of-life issues may be valued more by patients than the changes in medical risk often prioritised by practitioners.

Evaluation can vary at different times

Evaluation can take place at different stages of an intervention and this influences the information collected.

Example 1

When evaluating the impact of contacts at which the issue of obesity is raised, consider:

Patient's reaction to raising the issue

- When invited to discuss the issue of their weight, did the patient agree or decline?
- When raising the issue, to what extent did the practitioner use a nonjudgmental approach?

Extent of learning
To what extent did the patient improve knowledge and awareness of:

- The extent of their own weight problem?
- The consequences of overweight?
- The benefits of modest weight loss?
- The pros and cons of change?

Intention to change
If there was agreement to discuss weight, how did this influence the patient's intention to change?

- Not intending to take action
- Intending to take action in the future (next 6 months)
- Intending to make changes now
- Already making changes

Example 2

When evaluating the outcome of giving a leaflet on dietary changes for weight loss, consider:

Leaflet content

- Visual appeal of the written literature
- Suitability of language used
- Suitability of content for ethnic group
- Ease of understanding of the information

Extent of learning
To what extent did the patient improve knowledge and awareness of:

- Their own eating habits?
- How to make low-calorie foods choices?
- How to track progress?
- Common food sources of excess calories?
- Portion sizes?
- Meal preparation and food purchasing?

Example 3

When evaluating the outcome of a 6 month dietary treatment, consider:

Clinical information

- Weight, BMI, % weight loss (3, 6 months)
- Blood pressure (0, 3, 6 months)
- HbA1c and fasting glucose (0, 6 months)
- Lipid profile (0, 6 months)
- Vitamin D (0, 3 months)
- Binge-eating scores (0, 6 months)
- Behavioural changes: diet quality (0, 3, 6 months), regular eating (0, 3, 6 months), self-monitoring (0, 3, 6 months)

PROMs (Patient Reported Outcome Measures)

- Quality-of-life measures (0, 6 months)
- Symptom and functional changes (0, 6 months)

PREMs (Patient Reported Experience Measures)

- Satisfaction questionnaire (3, 6 months)
- Trust patient experience questionnaire

What makes evaluation challenging?

There are a number of difficulties which may explain why evaluation is often neglected. These include:

- Uncertainty about what to measure
- Uncertainty about the best tools with which to gather information
- Uncertainty and limited confidence in skills to undertake evaluation
- Perceived lack of time

Unstructured weight-management activities which are unclear about what they are trying to achieve can hinder evaluation. For example, activities with no formal goal-setting or inconsistent referral or discharge protocols make measuring the impact of weight management more challenging.

Evaluation in obesity is a 'work in progress'. More needs to be understood about the best outcome measures to use in order to capture the broad impact of lifestyle modification in obesity management. In particular, validated tools are needed which can be used in clinical practice, for example in relation to the assessment of dietary intake. For further information, refer to the National Obesity Observatories Standards for Weight Management [5] and the National American Association for the Study of Obesity Tools Project [6].

Traditionally, obesity evaluation has looked only at weight and BMI changes. Used alone, these are unlikely to capture the broader effects of treatment. Rather than just reflecting changes in clinical risk, outcomes need to consider the full impact on the physical, social, psychological and economic consequences of obesity. For example, weight management may have beneficial effects on self-esteem or aspects of quality of life independent of weight change.

Getting started

To begin the evaluation of a weight-management activity can seem daunting. The following suggestions may be helpful in starting the process:

1   Set up a planning meeting and develop clear aims and objectives for the weight-management activity/programme
2   Think through the patient, practitioner and commissioners needs in the evaluation as these will affect the information which needs to be collected
3   Decide on what information needs to be collected and how this will be done
4   Decide on the times at which information will be collected. For example, at baseline (before treatment), immediately after treatment, at 3 months, at 6 months and at 1 year
5   Decide on whether there are the skills and resources within the team with which to find, adapt or develop tools to collect information, interpret findings and/or write up a final report
6   Involve service users in the development of tools. This is important if genuine person-centredness is to be adopted. Patients need to be listened to and services improved according to their feedback
7   Use validated tools if they are available and are suitable for your local population
8   Consider amending an existing tool to the needs of your local population, with the permission of the author
9   Consider using a range of tools and don't be afraid to be creative and think outside the box
10   Identify additional resources or expertise if required
11   Gather baseline information at the first (assessment) consultation and collect follow-up information at a concluding appointment
12   Develop an assessment template that will help collect all required baseline information
13   Develop spreadsheets to help organise information collected

Collecting information

The information collected should be strongly linked to the overall aims and objectives of the weight-management activity. Once it is clear exactly what the 'activity' aims to achieve, the information that needs to be collected will become more obvious.

To some extent the way information is collected will depend on the time available and the level of expertise locally. It may be necessary to find specialist help if more complex methods of collecting information are chosen. If there are limited resources,either in time or expertise, keep information collected simple.

Where possible, choose a validated tool, so long as it is suitable for the local population and is not too time-consuming for the patient to complete or the practitioner to interpret.

There are a number of different approaches that can be used to collect information, including:

- questionnaires
- case studies
- interviews
- focus groups
- photographs

Questionnaires are probably the most popular strategy and typically explore opinions, attitudes and/or current practices. They are, however, limited by their reliance on self-reported information.

Before deciding to develop a new questionnaire, ensure there isn't one already available that would be suitable for the local population.

However, if it is necessary to develop a questionnaire, consider the following points:

1   What is the objective of the questionnaire?
2   Decide on a series of topics and then carefully plan questions to address those areas
3   How will it be administered (e.g. pen and paper completed by patient, Web based, etc.)?
4   Check all questions are relevant to the purpose of the questionnaire, to prevent it becoming too long and unclear
5   Include a mixture of different types of questions (open and closed), which will keep people interested and may expand on the views expressed
6   Pilot the questionnaire and check its readability and the time it takes to complete
7   If questionnaires are completed by staff, ensure this is done in a person-centred way. Convey genuine interest in the client's responses and use reflective listening skills, rather than just asking a series of questions

Open-ended questions

These allow people to express their views and ideas more freely, which may identify issues otherwise not considered.
Example: 'What aspect of the programme helped you most in making healthier food choices?'
Open-ended questions are often put towards the end of the questionnaire, which allows people time to settle into the subject before being asked to express their views more freely.

Closed questions

There are a variety of closed question styles, including:
Checklist (range of answers, with one or all that apply chosen)

Q: How often do you read food labels?
A: Every time I shop/Sometimes when I shop/I never read food labels

Scaled items (Strength of agreement/disagreement)

Q: I was treated with dignity and respect
A: Strongly agree/Agree/Neither agree nor disagree/Disagree/Strongly disagree

For further information on key tools, refer to 'Experienced Based Design' from the NHS Institute for Innovation and Improvement (http://www.institute.nhs.uk/quality_and_value/introduction/experience_based_design.html).

What to evaluate

Effectiveness

Being effective is about making a difference to clinical outcomes, identifying the quality of processes through clinical audit and ensuring practitioners are effective through staff training.

Clinical outcomes

Clearly, weight change is an important measure of effectiveness and patients are now encouraged to set modest 5–10% weight-loss targets over a 6 month period. Although some patients will achieve this amount of weight loss, others may not. Setting weight-change targets at the first consultation is important as it allows progress to be tracked and outcomes determined. For patients with more complex histories or with conditions such as type 2 diabetes, where weight loss is more difficult, lower targets may be appropriate (e.g. 0–3%). In those who have experienced a period of rapid weight gain, stabilisation of weight may be the chosen target. It is important to remember that although the weight-loss target for a weight-management service may be 5% over 6–9 months, there will be individual variation, and for some patients any weight loss will be an achievement.

Remember: with no treatment, weight usually increases by about 1 kg each year [7].

For every 1 kg body weight lost there is an average:

- 0.68 mm Hg fall in systolic blood pressure
- 0.34 mm Hg fall in diastolic blood pressure
- 2.28 mg/dL fall in serum cholesterol
- 0.9 mg/dL fall in LDL cholesterol
- 1.54 mg/dL fall in triglycerides
- 0.2 mmol fall in fasting plasma glucose

As exercise can lower abdominal fat without any loss of body weight, measuring change in waist circumference is valuable. Research suggests significant reductions in health risks are observed with waist changes of 5–10 cm [8].

For every 1 kg weight loss, waist circumference will change by about 1 cm.

Risk factors

Changes in lifestyle can have beneficial effects in health without changes in weight and this fact needs to be captured.

It is suggested that the following clinical parameters should be collected:

- cardiovascular risk factors: triglyceride, LDL-cholesterol, HDL-cholesterol
- blood pressure
- blood glucose

Activity and eating behaviours

Beneficial changes to eating and activity behaviours are precursors to weight loss and are important short-term outcomes. However, they are complex behaviours and their measurement is particularly challenging.

Physical activity

Measurement of physical activity can be done objectively and/or subjectively.

Objective measures
These include pedometers, which measure the number of steps taken, or physical-activity monitors (PAMs); cost may dictate choice. The number of steps taken each day can then be compared to recommended targets. For further details, check out http://www.nhs.uk/Livewell/loseweight/Pages/10000stepschallenge.aspx.

> **In brief**
>
> 1 Request patients wear a pedometer daily and record the number of steps each day for 7 days before any changes are put into place (baseline measurement)
> 2 Repeat this process after physical-activity changes are established (e.g. 3–6 months)
> 3 Calculate the average difference between daily steps taken at baseline and steps taken after intervention
> 4 Consider presenting information in a graphical format

These approaches are well validated, can be undertaken with limited burden to the patient and do not require accurate recording of activity behaviours. However, they do not provide information on the type of exercise chosen.

There are also Web sites which support tracking physical activity using GPS technology (e.g. Nike Plus or www.endomondo.com) and can support motivation in some clients.

Subjective measures

Measuring physical activity using questionnaires is common practice, although it is important to use high-quality tools. A recent review of tools available suggested the questionnaires below were validated for use in adults [9].

- Stanford 7-day Recall:
  - Leisure and recreational activity evaluated using an interview-administered questionnaire
  - Approximately 15 minutes to complete
  - A formula can be used to convert findings into kcal of energy expended.
  - Further details are available from http://www.drjamessallis.sdsu.edu/sevendayparprotocol.pdf (last accessed 22 August 2011)
- New Zealand Physical Activity Questionnaire:
  - Self-completion questionnaire
  - Approximately 10 minutes to complete
  - Suitable for adults age 40–79 years
  - Not commonly used in the UK
  - Further details are available from references [10] and [11]

Dietary intake

Changes to food choices which lead to changes in calorie intake are a key objective in weight management. However, demonstrating this change is challenging as measurement of dietary intake is complex and fraught with difficulties. The only tools currently available to use in clinical practice are self-report measures. Misreporting of calorie and fat intake is common and is more likely to occur in overweight and obese people. The 7-day weighed food diary is the most accurate measure but it involves a substantial amount of analysis for the practitioner. At present there is no simple validated tool for measuring dietary intake in the UK and this remains an ongoing challenge in demonstrating that nutrition interventions make a difference to dietary behaviours [5].

It may be helpful to consider some of the dietary issues below:

Regularity of meals

- Average number of times per week the patient eats breakfast
- Average number of times per week the patient eats lunch
- Average number of times per week the patient eats an evening meal

Eating out and/or takeaways

- Average number of times per week the patient eats out or has takeaway foods

Daily portions of fruit and vegetables eaten

- Average number of times a day the patient eats fruit
- Average number of times a day the patient eats vegetables

Sugary drinks

- Average number of times per week the patient has a sugary drink

For further information, check out references [9] and [12]

Also consider:

What are the nutritional goals of care agreed between patient and practitioner? To what extent have these goals been met?

- achieved
- partially achieved
- not achieved

Have any measured improvements to nutritional status occurred?

- e.g. vitamin D level

Changes in the quality of dietary intake can be assessed prior to the start of the programme and at various stages thereafter by taking reported daily portions from each of the food groups on the 'eatwell plate' (Tool 12) and comparing to the recommended intake.

Psychological health

Untreated depression and anxiety may make obesity management and changing lifestyle more challenging than usual. As such, it may be useful to screen people for risk of depression and anxiety and refer for further support from the GP or mental health team if scores suggest further intervention would be merited. This may mean obesity treatment is delayed until mood can be stabilised and the patient is in a better place psychologically to begin to think about making changes to diet and physical-activity behaviours.

PHQ-9 [13] is a quick tool used in primary care to determine risk of depression (further information can be obtained from http://www.depression-primarycare. org/clinicians/toolkits/materials/forms/phq9/). GAD 7 is a quick tool for assessing anxiety [14].

Health care utilisation and cost outcomes

Obesity significantly increases health care costs, particularly drug prescription costs [15]. Therefore, investing in weight management has the potential to reduce the costs of care for obese patients in primary care.

Counterweight, an obesity-management primary care programme, found men with a BMI between 25 and 30 had annual drug prescription costs £7.78 higher for every 1 unit increase in BMI; for women costs were £5.53 higher. This effect was even greater when the top 10 most popular drugs were considered.

> Minimum annual drug costs at BMI 20 were £50.71 in men and £62.59 in women. Minimum annual drug costs at BMI 40 were £198.66 in men and £160.73 in women. 16% of the total prescribing costs in primary care can be attributed to obesity and 26% to overweight and obesity [16].

Given the potential to decrease spending on drug prescribing and health care utilisation generally, it is important to record certain economic factors. These may include:

- Medication changes (brand, strength, no tablets/ml before and after treatment)
- Number of inpatient days
- Number of outpatient days
- Planned/unplanned clinic visits

Patient experience

A true commitment to patient-centred care demands careful consideration of the patient's views on treatment outcomes and experiences and the incorporation of these findings into future services. Patient views on their experience of receiving treatment (referred to as PREMs) are the primary source of information.

Patient-reported experience measures (PREMs)

Understanding more about what matters most to patients.

PREMs, together with routinely reported complaints and compliments, provide important perspectives on a patient's experience of treatment and insight into what they believe makes a high-quality service. This allows best practice and lessons learnt to be fed back to other members of the team so care can be improved.

So, for example, PREMs might highlight poor access to a weight-management clinic and the need to redesign the appointment system.

PREMs might include a rating of overall experience followed more specifically by aspects such as:

- Politeness, dignity, respect
- Convenience and timing of appointments
- Appropriateness of the clinic environment
- Understandability of information presented
- Listening skills of the practitioner
- Patient involvement in the weight-management plan
- Continuity of care

Satisfaction generally occurs when the patient's perceptions of care match their expectations. Various factors are believed to influence satisfaction, including professional care, the depth of the patient/practitioner relationship and the perceived adequacy of time provided [17].

Questionnaires to assess a patient's experience of treatment can be administered at different time points and questions tailored accordingly. For example, after the first appointment they might include questions such as:

- I was satisfied with the information I received before this appointment
- I was aware of how many sessions were being offered and how these would be structured
- I felt I had a chance to tell the story about my weight
- I felt the practitioner was nonjudgmental during the consultation
- I found the seating comfortable
- I was aware of how to contact the practitioner if there were any difficulties before my next appointment

(Strongly agree/Agree/Neither disagree nor agree/Disagree/Strongly disagree.)

The patient's experience can then be evaluated throughout their journey from the referral to the first outpatient consultation and beyond the treatment stage to discharge. Also, general questions relating to patients experience of treatment can be administered at the end of the treatment period.

Example questions

Responses would use a five-point Likert scale:

Strongly agree/Agree/Neither disagree nor agree/Disagree/Strongly disagree.

1   Overall I felt satisfied with the weight-management service I received
2   I felt I was listened to by the practitioner
3   I was involved in developing my weight-management plan

> 4   The information I was given was helpful
> 5   The appointments generally took place on time
> 6   I could generally see the same practitioner at each appointment
> 7   I was treated with dignity and respect
> 8   I was given enough privacy during weight checks
> 9   I trusted the practitioner who treated me
> 10 I would recommend this weight-management service to others

Targets can be set locally, against which measures can be compared. So, for example, it may be decided that the target is for 80% of patients to respond 'Agree' or 'Strongly agree' to the question on overall experience of treatment.

Questionnaires are often used to collect PREMs. Interviews and focus groups may be used but tend to be more time-intensive. It is critical that patients are involved in the development of measurement tools in order to ensure the content truly reflects the patient's rather than the practitioner's priorities.

Further information on designing a patient-centred questionnaire can be obtained from reference [18].

Patient-reported outcome measures (PROMs)

PROMs are important in helping practitioners understand the impact of obesity on the patient's life, and the effectiveness of treatment from the patient's perspective. This information can be very valuable in the design and development of weight-management services.

PROMs tend to cover three broad areas:

- **Quality of life**   Overall rating of satisfaction with life
- **Symptoms linked with obesity**   Shortness of breath, fatigue, joint pain, sleeping difficulties
- **Changes in function linked with obesity**   Difficulties with self care, e.g. washing, dressing

Weight management may improve symptoms such as shortness of breath or sleeping difficulties, or improve the patient's ability to socialise through improved self-esteem. Measuring these areas alongside clinical outcomes is therefore important. There are very few validated tools which have been developed to measure these outcomes in obese people. However, it has been suggested that the symptom assessment scale shown in Table 11.1 could be adapted for use in obesity.

There are also a number of general tools that measure health-related quality of life which include aspects of function and could easily be modified using the phrase 'because of your obesity':

- EQ-5D-5L (www.euroqol.org)
- SF-36 (www.sf36.com)

Table 11.1 Symptom status: example of adapting the Memorial Symptom Assessment Scale for obesity [14]

Instructions: We have listed eight symptoms below. Read each one carefully. If you have had the symptom during the past 3 months, let us know how OFTEN you had it, how SEVERE it was usually, and how much it DISTRESSED or BOTHERED you by circling the appropriate number. If you DID NOT HAVE the symptom, make an X in the box marked DID NOT HAVE.

DURING THE PAST THREE MONTHS, Did you have any of the following symptoms?	Did not have	IF YES, How often did you have it?				IF YES, How SEVERE is it usually?				IF YES, How much did it DISTRESS or BOTHER you?				
		Rarely	Occasionally	Frequently	Almost constantly	Slight	Moderate	Severe	Very severe	Not at all	A little bit	Somewhat	Quite a bit	Very much
Low back pain	☐	1	2	3	4	1	2	3	4	0	1	2	3	4
Joint pain or stiffness (including hips, knees & back)	☐	1	2	3	4	1	2	3	4	0	1	2	3	4
Shortness of breath or difficulty breathing	☐	1	2	3	4	1	2	3	4	0	1	2	3	4
General fatigue, tiredness, weakness	☐	1	2	3	4	1	2	3	4	0	1	2	3	4
Chest pain, pressure, palpitations or other discomfort in the chest	☐	1	2	3	4	1	2	3	4	0	1	2	3	4
Sleep disturbance	☐	1	2	3	4	1	2	3	4	0	1	2	3	4
Anxiety	☐	1	2	3	4	1	2	3	4	0	1	2	3	4
Depression	☐	1	2	3	4	1	2	3	4	0	1	2	3	4

Alternatively, the IWQOL-Lite is a validated quality-of-life tool specifically designed for use in the obese population [19]. There is a fee for its use in clinical practice; further details are available at http://www.qualityoflifeconsulting.com/iwqol-lite.html.

Safety

Evaluating safety requires a system of routine reporting of safety-related incidents, and particularly of near misses, to ensure lessons can be learnt and strategies are put in place to prevent future events. This will only be possible in a culture of openness and with a commitment to learning from experience.

Key safety themes may include:

- Well being of patients and staff
- Communication (particularly relating to referrals)
- Violence and abuse of staff

Monitoring of incidents, near misses and complaints may highlight issues such as:

- Inadequate information provided by a referrer
- Failure of staff to meet work dress code
- Unsafe chairs or inadequate weighing equipment
- Weighing of patients in the reception area, with limited privacy
- Poor meet-and-greet at the reception area
- Inadequate training of staff on conflict resolution
- Poor storage of records

This will highlight issues which need to be addressed and identify potential training requirements.

Conclusion

Evaluation is essential to our understanding of the quality of lifestyle treatments in the management of obesity, not just in terms of clinical outcomes, but importantly in those results and experiences most valued by patients. Through broadening the outcome measures used we can capture the multifaceted treatment effect of lifestyle modification and use these findings for the continued development of the quality of interventions and services.

If evaluation seems daunting, keep data collection simple in the early stages and expand as your confidence grows.

Consider this

- Are you currently collecting data?
- If not, what would need to happen to achieve this?
- Who would you need to speak to for further help?
- Does your assessment template/tool facilitate the collection of baseline information?

References

1. Appleby J, Ham C, Imison C, Jennings M. Improving NHS productivity. More with the same not more of the same. The Kings Fund; 2010.
2. Schmadl JC. Quality assurance: examination of the concept. Nursing Outlook 1979;27[7]:462–5.
3. Sale D, editor. Understanding Clinical Governance and Quality Assurance: Making it Happen Basingstoke: Palgrave Macmillan; 2005.
4. Royal College of Physicians. The Training of Health Professionals for the Prevention and Treatment of Overweight and Obesity. Royal College of Physicians; 2010.
5. National Obesity Observatory. Standard Evaluation Framework for Weight Management Interventions. National Obesity Observatory; 2009.
6. Wolf AM. Task Force on Developing Obesity Outcomes and Learning Standards Obesity Research. Obesity Research 2002;10:1S–2S.
7. Lewis CE, Jacobs DR, Jr, McCreath H, Kiefe CI, Schreiner PJ, Smith DE, et al. Weight gain continues in the 1990s: 10-year trends in weight and overweight from the CARDIA study. Coronary Artery Risk Development in Young Adults. Am J Epidemiol 2000 Jun 15;151[12]:1172–81.
8. Aronne LJ, Segal KR. Adiposity and fat distribution outcome measures: assessment and clinical implications. Obes Res 2002 Nov;10[Suppl. 1]:14S–21S.
9. National Obesity Observatory. Measuring Diet and Physical Activity in Weight Management Interventions. National Obesity Observatory; 2011.
10. Maddison R, Ni Mhurchu C, Jiang Y, Vander Hoorn S, Rodgers A, Lawes CM, et al. International Physical Activity Questionnaire (IPAQ) and New Zealand Physical Activity Questionnaire (NZPAQ): a doubly labelled water validation. Int J Behav Nutr Phys Act 2007;4:62.
11. Lawton BA, Rose SB, Elley CR, Dowell AC, Fenton A, Moyes SA. Exercise on prescription for women aged 40–74 recruited through primary care: two year randomised controlled trial. BMJ 2008;337:a2509.
12. Gans KM, Ross E, Barner CW, Wylie-Rosett J, McMurray J, Eaton C. REAP and WAVE: new tools to rapidly assess/discuss nutrition with patients. J Nutr 2003 Feb;133[2]:556S–62S.
13. Kroenke K, Spitzer RL, Williams JB. The PHQ-9: validity of a brief depression severity measure. J Gen Intern Med 2001 Sep;16[9]:606–13.
14. Spitzer RL, Kroenke K, Williams JB, Lowe B. A brief measure for assessing generalized anxiety disorder: the GAD-7. Arch Intern Med 2006 May 22;166[10]:1092–7.
15. National Obesity Observatory. The Economic Burden of Obesity. National Obesity Observatory; 2010.
16. Counterweight Project Team. Influence of body mass index on prescribing costs and potential cost savings of a weight management programme in primary care. Journal of Health Services Research & Policy 2008;13[3]:158–66.
17. Crow R, Storey L, Page H. The measurement of patient satisfaction: implications for health services delivery through a systematic review of the conceptual, methodological and empirical literature. Health Technology Assessment 2003;6[32].
18. Reay N. How to measure patient experience and outcomes to demonstrate quality in care. Nurs Times 2010 Feb 23–Mar 1;106[7]:12–4.
19. Kolotkin RL, Crosby RD. Psychometric evaluation of the impact of weight on quality of life-lite questionnaire (IWQOL-lite) in a community sample. Qual Life Res 2002 Mar;11[2]:157–71.

12 Common Challenges and Misconceptions

'Challenges are what make life interesting, overcoming them is what makes life meaningful.'

Joshua J. Marne

Introduction

Patient consultations provide a number of challenges for practitioners to address, not only in maintaining up-to-date knowledge of the latest evidence but also in having the communication skills to deliver this information in a supportive and helpful way. A number of common challenges are addressed in this chapter.

Causes of obesity

'It's my fault I'm obese'

Background

It's unsurprising given the widespread negative attitudes to obesity that patients often blame themselves for their size. There is a commonly held notion that obesity is a self-inflicted condition which results from irresponsible food and activity choices and that the only person to blame is the obese individual. This can be damaging to self-esteem and is not a good platform from which to consider implementing changes to lifestyle.

Evidence

As outlined in Chapter 1, obesity is caused by a complex mix of genetic and environmental factors, the contribution and relevance of which varies from one individual to another [1]. Given the range of environmental factors involved, it follows that there are social and corporate responsibilities as well as personal ones. If the environment promotes obesity, as it certainly does, people will gain weight,

Weight Management: A Practitioner's Guide, First Edition. Dympna Pearson and Clare Grace.
© 2012 Dympna Pearson and Clare Grace. Published 2012 by Blackwell Publishing Ltd.

particularly those who are genetically predisposed. A more positive approach is to move away from a culture of self-blame towards developing an environment where healthier choices are easier, and those who struggle to control their weight also acknowledge that lifestyle change can make a difference to weight-loss outcomes (though these remain an ongoing challenge).

Patient dialogue

Patient: *'It's terrible to think that I let myself get to this size! It's my own fault, I just can't say "no" to nice food. I feel mortified!*

Practitioner: *'You feel bad about how your weight has increased.'*

Patient: *'Yes, it's entirely my fault – I know that's what everyone thinks. But I just have no willpower! I hate being this size so much that you would think that I would be able to follow a diet.'*

Practitioner: *'You sound really down about it. Many people who struggle with their weight say similar things. Am I right that you would really like to lose weight but you are not sure if you can?*

Patient: *'Exactly! I would give anything to be a normal size, but I just can't stop eating.'*

Practitioner: *'It sounds as if you are blaming yourself and as a result feeling even worse, which means you find it even harder to follow a diet?'*

Patient: *'Yes, no matter how hard I try…'*

Practitioner: *'I think you are being very hard on yourself. People put weight on for a whole variety of reasons and living in today's world doesn't make it easy to avoid high-calorie foods. It can be especially difficult for people like yourself who have always struggled with their weight. Developing the skills to say "no" is something that is entirely possible and we can think about how you can best do that.'*

Patient: *'So you don't think I am a hopeless case then!'*

'I must have a slow metabolism'

Background

There is a widely held belief that obese people have a slow metabolism and this is a cause of overweight. Linked with this belief is the idea that some obese people eat next to nothing and still gain weight. In a few rare instances, weight gain can be explained by a medical condition, and this needs to be ruled out by a medical practitioner. For the majority, the issues below are more relevant.

Evidence

'Metabolic rate' describes the calories used by the body to keep basic bodily systems functioning. This is often called 'resting metabolic rate' and makes up a substantial proportion of total calories expended, particularly in people who are sedentary. For years, scientists were baffled by individuals who reported eating next to nothing but still gaining weight. They searched for possible biological explanations but no studies have found obese people with abnormally low metabolic rates. Indeed, the amount of calories obese people need to keep their bodies functioning is generally higher than for an average-weight person [2]. This is because as weight is gained there is an increase not only in fat tissue but also in muscle mass, and it this latter component that plays a major part in determining metabolic rate. The higher the muscle mass, the higher the metabolic rate and the more energy the body will use up each day.

Patient dialogue

Patient: *'I must have a slow metabolism. I mean, I just can't lose weight, no matter what I eat!'*
Practitioner: *'You think your metabolism is causing you not to lose weight.'*
Patient: *'Yes, well, I hardly eat a thing and I still can't lose!'*
Practitioner: *'Even though you eat very little, the weight still doesn't come off.'*
Patient: *'That's right, I have more or less given up because nothing works.'*
Practitioner: *'You sound totally disheartened by the whole thing. Would you like me to explain what is known about how metabolism affects weight?'*
Patient: *'OK.'*
Practitioner: *'People used to think that metabolism was the cause of a lot of weight problems and because of that, a lot of research has been done in this area. It has been found that metabolism doesn't play such a big role. When someone isn't losing weight, science tells us that they are taking in more calories than **their** body needs. What seems most helpful is to focus on specific aspects of eating and activity. Are you happy to consider that?'*

'It's my genes, not my lifestyle'

Background

This is sometimes perceived by practitioners as an excuse used by patients to avoid acknowledging the reality of their eating and activity behaviours. However, the evidence tells us something very different.

Evidence

Family studies have shown that obesity is strongly influenced by genetics. Until recently, only serious genetic mutations that cause rare obesity syndromes such as Prader–Willi or Bardet–Biedl syndrome had been identified. Finding common genes that might play a part in explaining why large numbers of obese people struggle to control their weight remained elusive until recently. A specific gene, called FTO, has now been identified which increases the risk of obesity and affects about one in six people [3]. Although this is important in terms of understanding more about how weight is regulated, at present it doesn't change available treatments offered or the need to focus on lifestyle management. Those that are predisposed to overweight and obesity will need to be more vigilant than others and consciously control their lifestyle behaviours [4].

Patient dialogue

Patient: *'I think it's my genes. I mean, all my family are overweight and I just can't lose weight no matter how hard I try!'*
Practitioner: *'You think your genes are causing your weight problem.'*
Patient: *'Yes, I read an article about it in the paper the other day and I think I am just one of those people who can't lose no matter what they try.'*
Practitioner: *'You sound very frustrated with your experience of your weight-loss efforts.'*
Patient: *'Yeah, I just think, "What's the point?"'*
Practitioner: *'Would you like me to explain what is known about the part that genes play?'*
Patient: *'Yes!'*
Practitioner: *'It has been found that genes do make some people more susceptible to weight gain, and in turn they find it harder to lose weight than others.'*
Patient: *'I knew it!'*
Practitioner: *'So that confirms your experience. The good news from the research that has been done is that it is still possible to lose weight even if you have the "wrong set of genes". It means that you have to work hard at making changes to eating and activity and it may take longer than you would like, but it is possible and I am happy to support you if you would like to persevere.'*
Patient: *'Well, if I know I have support, that will help.'*

'I've been told I'm not eating enough to lose weight'

Background

Patients sometimes believe their struggle to lose weight may be because they are not eating enough. This may occur when patients fail to lose weight while reporting a very low calorie intake. It is sometimes questioned whether such patients are in 'starvation mode', where the body tries to conserve body fat by becoming increasingly energy-efficient. Sometimes patients are told to eat 'more' to help them lose weight, but this message can be very confusing and there are a number of issues that need to be clarified.

Evidence

If a person isn't losing weight, their energy intake must exceed their expenditure [5]. For example, a 100 kg 45-year-old male patient reporting an intake of 800 calories/day with no accompanying weight loss must be underestimating their intake as their daily calorie requirements are approximately 2600 calories to maintain their weight. Given how challenging it is to recall/record food intake, it isn't surprising that under-reporting of calorie intake is common. Patients may also be concerned they will be judged for their reported intake and so consciously or unconsciously are reluctant to reveal the reality of their eating (see more about accurate recording of food intake in Chapter 7). So if a person's weight is static, they must be eating the same number of calories as their body is using, or if their weight is increasing, calories eaten must be greater than those used up. The message that a person isn't eating enough is inaccurate and very unhelpful in this situation. In most instances, support is needed to unpick the aspects of lifestyle leading to the excess calorie intake.

It is true that foods protective against obesity (e.g. fruits and vegetables, wholegrain foods) may not be eaten in sufficient quantities while those which promote obesity (e.g. high-sugar drinks, high-calorie snack foods) may be eaten in too great an amount. However, this requires a shift in the balance of foods eaten or a change of portion sizes, rather than a blanket message that an inadequate amount is being eaten.

There is an interesting question about whether as someone cuts down their calorie intake it slows down metabolism, thereby preventing further weight loss. It is this response to 'dieting' which is sometimes blamed for the challenge of continued weight loss. Although the body does adapt and become more metabolically efficient as calorie intake is reduced, the effect is not large, and is unlikely to account for the difficulties people experience. Metabolic rate drops by about 5% (on intakes ~1200 kcal/day), much less than is imagined by many patients and practitioners. Even on a very-low-calorie diet of <800 calories/day, metabolic rate falls by no more than 15% [6]. Although this will make some difference to the number of calories someone will be able to eat before weight is gained, it is not the primary explanation for the difficulties with continued weight loss.

Patient dialogue

Patient: 'The last person I saw said I must not be eating enough!'
Practitioner: 'Many people believe that can explain when someone who is trying hard doesn't lose weight.'
Patient: 'Do you think that is the case with me?'
Practitioner: 'Would you like me to explain what I understand about this?'
Patient: 'OK.'
Practitioner: 'It seems that there is no getting away from the calories in/calories out equation. What is now understood is how very difficult it is to estimate the calories we take in. Research that has looked at how accurate people are when they report or record what they eat has found that we can underestimate our intake by as much 50% [7]. It is virtually impossible to be 100% accurate in estimating our calorie intake. Even small inaccuracies in our recording or reporting of foods eaten can be the difference between losing and not losing weight. Is this something you would like to know more about?'
Patient: 'I guess so.'
Practitioner: 'It seems that success lies in becoming a "food detective" and putting a lot of effort into tracking your food intake.'
Patient: 'You mean keeping a diary?' [See Chapter 7.]

Physical activity

'I can't lose weight because my medical problems stop me from exercising'

Background

There are medical consequences of obesity which may interfere with a patient's ability to adopt healthier lifestyle choices and which contribute to further weight gain. Knee, back and joint problems may be exacerbated by obesity and make engaging in substantial amounts of physical activity very challenging, if not impossible. Likewise, poorly controlled obstructive sleep apnoea may produce levels of sleepiness and fatigue that erode people's resolve to change behaviour. Depression can interfere with motivation, energy and perceived capacity to change. Poor sleep, pain, fatigue, low mood and lack of energy are not the best starting place for creating and sustaining change.

Evidence

Ensuring the medical condition has received the best possible care prior to starting a weight-management attempt is very important. Treatment for certain conditions may be delayed assuming weight loss will improve the symptoms, or a clear diagnosis may be not be sought prior to beginning a weight-loss programme. However, poor sleep, pain, fatigue and low mood interfere with a person's ability to begin, and sustain, changes to lifestyle. As such, weight-loss outcomes and symptom improvement are likely to be poorer. Treating depression or sleep apnoea, for example, before the start of a programme may place the person in a better position from which to invest the time and energy needed to change lifestyle choices over the long term [8].

Patient dialogue

Patient: '*I can't lose weight because I can't do any exercise. My knee is really painful – it's just hopeless!*'
Practitioner: '*You are sounding disheartened about your weight because of the difficulties with your knee.*'
Patient: '*Yes, the doctor said I had to lose 3 stones but there is no way I can do that!*'
Practitioner: '*I can see that you are totally daunted at the prospect of trying to lose that amount, especially when you are hampered by your knee pain. Would you like to discuss what I think is possible?*'
Patient: '*You mean there is some hope for me?*'
Practitioner: '*Yes. I think it is important to be realistic about the amount of weight that it is possible for you to lose, but even half a stone is likely to take some pressure off your knee. Second, for weight loss to happen, food plays a bigger part during the weight-loss phase, and although activity is also important, it really comes into its own when trying to keep any weight you lose off over the long term. How about if we focus initially on the food side of things and then hopefully, if your knee pain improves, we can think about the activity side?*'
Patient: '*OK, that makes sense.*'

'Exercise makes me eat more'

Background

There is debate about whether the body compensates for the extra energy used during exercise by increasing hunger (and food intake) to protect against the loss of body fat. Increased hunger is often reported by patients, but is this reality or misperception?

Evidence

Research suggests acute bouts of exercise do not increase hunger [9], the desire to eat or energy intake, but the impact of regular exercise over the long term is less clear [10]. Most studies conclude moderate activity does not increase hunger in overweight and obese individuals, although individual variation in weight-loss response to exercise is recognised [11]. The reasons why some people respond poorly to exercise are not well understood but are likely to be a complex mix of physiological, psychological and behavioural factors. One way in which being active may lead to increased energy intake is through an increased sense of entitlement to eat favourite high-calorie foods. It is not uncommon to use food-based rewards after exercise (e.g. having a chocolate bar or drink from the vending machine after swimming) as a way of acknowledging the successful completion of an activity goal without realising the misjudgements that may be being made [12]. So it is useful to help patients think through their eating habits in relation to activity and how they may be undermining their weight-management attempts.

Patient dialogue

Patient: *'Exercise makes me eat more – I'm always starving after I get home from the gym.'*
Practitioner: *'A lot of people say that they feel hungrier after exercise.'*
Patient: *'It's not just me then?'*
Practitioner: *'Are you interested in knowing more about this?'*
Patient: *'It feels pretty pointless exercising if it causes me to eat more.'*
Practitioner: *'It seems that the need or desire for food is caused by a number of things and working out which one is relevant for you can be helpful. It is also worth considering what you mean by hunger. Sometimes what we believe is hunger may be food cravings and can be linked with certain activities or feelings [see Chapter 8]. Sometimes, we feel we deserve a reward after all that hard work and head for the vending machine or the bar! Sometimes people don't want to eat before exercise and end up going for long periods without food and then find themselves over-hungry after exercise and consequently over-eat. The secret might be to have a snack before exercise. There are many possibilities, which is why it is a good idea to track what happens for you. Would you be happy to do that?'*
Patient: *'Yes, I want to get this sorted.'*

'I've been swimming for 20 minutes twice a week for 2 months and haven't lost any weight'

Background

It is not uncommon for patients to remark that regular activity has had little impact on weight loss. This often relates to misunderstandings about the role of physical activity in the management of weight and the difficulty of losing weight through changes to activity alone. Alternatively, it can reflect an overestimation of calories used during exercise.

Evidence

Swimming at a constant pace for 20 minutes will burn off approximately 200–300 calories, depending on body size. If no other changes to lifestyle or eating occur, it will take 6–9 weeks of 20 minutes' swimming twice a week to produce a 0.5 kg weight loss. On the other hand, it is very easy to replace all these calories by eating, for example, one average-sized chocolate bar. It may also be physically impossible for some individuals to undertake this amount of activity in the early stages of managing their weight, when fitness or functional ability may be limited. The level of activity achievable in these instances would have a lesser effect on weight loss per se. In such situations, people may conclude the effort required outweighs the potential benefits. However, this underestimates the many positive health benefits associated with regular activity independent of weight loss, as well as its important effect on mood and self-esteem. The effect of exercise in helping people feel better about themselves may be critical to improving people's resolve to make and sustain changes to eating behaviours.

Patient dialogue

Patient: 'All that effort with swimming and it doesn't seem to make much difference – the weight should be dropping off me!'

Practitioner: 'It feels like you are putting in a lot of effort for very little return.'

Patient: 'Yes, exactly!'

Practitioner: 'I think it would be worth spending a few minutes discussing that. Would that be useful for you?'

Patient: 'Yes, OK.'

Practitioner: 'It's great that you have taken up swimming and your overall health will be benefitting. It is not uncommon for people to think the extra effort will make a big difference to weight loss – it certainly can feel like it! During this phase of your weight-management programme, exercise won't make a big difference to weight loss itself. Food plays a bigger part at this stage. However, every calorie counts and swimming, along with being as active as you can on a daily basis, adds to the calories your body uses up. The big benefits are to your overall health and to the "feel-good" effect of doing any exercise. Experts reckon that helps people keep to the diet side of things much better. How does that sound?'

Patient: 'OK, so I will keep up with the swimming, then.'

Diet

'Certain foods can burn fat'

Background

Do some foods have fat-burning properties that can speed up the metabolism and have beneficial effects on weight loss? Or is this just too good to be true? Citrus fruits, celery, green tea, cabbage and chillies are just a few examples of the foods sometimes cited as having fat-burning potential.

Evidence

There are no foods which burn body fat. Loss of body fat will only occur when the number of calories used up is greater than the number taken in from food. Although there are some foods which are higher in caffeine and this may temporarily raise metabolism, the effect is short-lived and insufficient to produce weight loss [13].

Patient dialogue

Patient: *'Is it true that certain foods burn fat? You know, grapefruit for example. And other foods have a negative calorie value like celery?'*
Practitioner: *'It sounds as if you are interested in getting your facts straight?'*
Patient: *'You hear so much, it starts to get confusing. I mean, the experts seem to keep changing their minds!'*
Practitioner: *'I agree it can be confusing with so much in the media these days about food. Unfortunately, not all of it is reliable and this is very frustrating for us as practitioners as well, especially as we have to make sure that any advice that we give is based on sound evidence.'*
Patient: *'So what are the good foods, then?'*
Practitioner: *'To be honest, it isn't that helpful to label foods as "good" and "bad". It is much more important to focus on the total calories in versus total calories out and try to aim for a healthy, balanced diet. And to answer your question, grapefruit doesn't burn fat and celery doesn't provide negative calories.'*
Patient: *'Oh well, thanks for clearing that up!'*

'I know breakfast is important but I just can't eat in the morning'

Background

Avoiding breakfast due to lack of appetite is a common reason cited for irregular eating. Is breakfast really that important and does the timing of breakfast really matter?

Evidence

There is increasing evidence to support the importance of including breakfast as part of a weight-management programme. Skipping breakfast has been associated with an increased risk of obesity and people who have successfully managed to lose large amounts of weight and maintain this loss are more likely to be regular breakfast-eaters [14]. Regular breakfast consumption may be beneficial through its influence on reducing impulsive snacking and reducing food intake at subsequent meals [15] (see Chapter 8). Exploring barriers to breakfast consumption can be helpful. Commonly cited difficulties are lack of time and lack of hunger, but a problem-solving approach can identify possible solutions. It is also worth highlighting that the timing of breakfast is not particularly important and it will remain beneficial whether it is eaten at 6 am or 10 am.

Patient dialogue

Patient: '*I just can't face breakfast in the mornings!*'
Practitioner: '*You are not a breakfast person.*'
Patient: '*No, it makes me feel sick!*' **or** '*If I have breakfast I can't stop eating all day. Surely I can save some calories if I skip breakfast?*'
Practitioner: '*You said you know breakfast is important. Would you like some additional information from the States about the benefits of breakfast for weight loss?*'
Patient: '*Yes.*'
Practitioner: '*They have collected data from over 10 000 people who have lost 30 lb [13.6 kg] or more and kept it off. They are keen to see whether these people have certain habits in common and having breakfast is one of them.*'
Patient: '*I guess if it works for that many people I had better give it a go. Would a banana count?*'
Practitioner: '*Absolutely, anything that "breaks the fast". We can look at this in more detail if you wish?*'
Patient: '*Yes, please. I'm really stuck for ideas!*'

'Carbs are fattening'

Background

It has been suggested that high-carbohydrate foods increase the likelihood of weight gain and this has fuelled the popularity of low-carbohydrate diets. It is usually the practitioner's role to provide some perspective on concepts such as 'all carbohydrates are fattening'.

Evidence

Many starchy foods, like bread, potatoes, rice and pasta, are naturally low in fat and calories. It is only through the addition of high-fat toppings or sauces that naturally healthy high-carbohydrate foods can be overloaded with calories.

Low-carbohydrate, high-protein diets have proved a popular weight-loss approach, although their efficacy and safety remain controversial. In the short term they do seem to produce greater weight loss, although by 1 year this difference has disappeared [16]. There are concerns about the relatively unknown effects of these diets on cardiovascular health, renal function, bone health and cancer risk, especially in those with obesity-related diseases, and there is evidence of nutritional shortfalls. There is interest in the potential for substituting a proportion of dietary energy from carbohydrate for protein while retaining a low fat intake. However, these approaches are different from the popular high-protein diets, being lower in protein (~25%E), much lower in fat (<30%E) and higher in carbohydrate (~40%). Early research suggests this approach may be beneficial in the short term [17], although beyond 1 year major benefits seem to be lost and there is a need for more research before amendments to advice occur (see more on evidence in Chapter 3).

Patient dialogue

Patient: *'I try not to eat carbs – they are fattening!'*
Practitioner: *'You are trying to avoid fattening foods.'*
Patient: *'Yes, I'm really keen to get rid of this weight!'*
Practitioner: *'Would it be OK if I share my concerns about avoiding carbohydrates?'*
Patient: *'OK, but I know it works – my friend tried it and lost loads of weight.'*
Practitioner: *'You are absolutely right that it is a very effective way of losing weight, especially in the short term. What we don't know are the long-term effects on your heart, kidney, bones and cancer risk. Also, although people lose weight quickly to begin with, at the end of a year the results show no difference in weight loss from following a healthy, balanced diet. I am keen to think about your overall health. What are your thoughts?'*
Patient: *'You mean I can still enjoy my pasta!'*

'Eating late at night causes weight gain'

Background

There is a commonly held view that eating late at night leads to greater weight gain than eating earlier in the day.

Evidence

A calorie is a calorie at any time of day and the body does not metabolise food differently depending on the time of day [18]. It is the total number of calories and the amount of activity taken in the day which makes the difference and affects weight. If too many calories are consumed then the body will store them as body fat, regardless of when they were eaten. However, many people who eat late at night tend to choose snack foods which are high in calories and eating at this time of day may be linked with boredom, stress, tiredness or situations such as watching television. Or it may be that larger portions are eaten if there have been long periods between meals. Therefore, although the time of day per se does not make a difference to the storage of excess calories, eating late at night can reflect eating and snacking habits that are likely to be linked with higher overall calorie intake.

Patient dialogue

Patient: *'I know eating late at night is bad, but I don't get home until late!'*
Practitioner: *'You are concerned that eating late at night will make it difficult for you to lose weight.'*
Patient: *'Yes, I read somewhere that you shouldn't eat after 6 pm!'*
Practitioner: *'It seems to be much more important **what** you eat rather than **when** you eat. People with busy lifestyles often struggle with mealtimes and it is advisable to try to spread your food intake throughout the day rather than have one big meal in the evening. Would you be happy to look at how your food fits into your day in more detail?'*
Patient: *'OK.'* [See examples of a typical day in Chapter 6, or encourage patient to keep a food diary (Chapter 7).]

Note on patient dialogues

The examples use reflective listening skills to deal with challenges. When patients say something that we disagree with or is clearly untrue, the temptation is to immediately disagree. This can cause needless conflict in the consultation and lead to the patient not feeling heard or understood. However, it is important that incorrect information or beliefs are clarified in a respectful way, by 'providing information in a helpful way' (see Chapter 7).

Consider this

- What situations do you find challenging in weight-management consultation?
- How do you react in those situations?
- Is there anything you could do differently?
- Remember that when consultations go badly, the temptation is to blame the patient. Reflective practice encourages us to consider our own attitude and our style of communicating.

References

1. Butland B, Jebb S, Kopelman P, McPherson K, Thomas S, Mardell J, Parry V. Foresight Tackling Obesities: Future Choices – Project Report. London: Government Office for Science; 2007.
2. Prentice AM, Black AE, Coward WA, Davies HL, Goldberg GR, Murgatroyd PR, et al. High levels of energy expenditure in obese women. Br Med J (Clin Res Ed) 1986 Apr 12;292[6526]:983–7.
3. Frayling TM, Timpson NJ, Weedon MN, Zeggini E, Freathy RM, Lindgren CM, et al. A common variant in the FTO gene is associated with body mass index and predisposes to childhood and adult obesity. Science 2007 May 11;316[5826]:889–94.
4. Loos RJ, Bouchard C. FTO: the first gene contributing to common forms of human obesity. Obes Rev 2008 May;9[3]:246–50.
5. Prentice AM. Obesity and its potential mechanistic basis. Br Med Bull 2001;60:51–67.
6. Prentice AM, Goldberg GR, Jebb SA, Black AE, Murgatroyd PR, Diaz EO. Physiological responses to slimming. Proc Nutr Soc 1991 Aug;50[2]:441–58.
7. Lichtman SW, Pisarska K, Berman ER, Pestone M, Dowling H, Offenbacher E, Weisel H, Heshka S, Matthews DE, Heymsfield SB. Discrepancy between self-reported and actual caloric intake and exercise in obese subjects. N Engl J Med 1992;327:1893–8.
8. Gregory SE, Rohde P, Ludman E, Jeffrey RW, Linde JA, Operskalski M, Arterburn D. Association between change in depression and change in weight among women enrolled in weight loss treatment. General Hospital Psychiatry 2010;32[6].
9. Unick JL, Otto AD, Goodpaster BH, Helsel DL, Pellegrini CA, Jakicic JM. Acute effect of walking on energy intake in overweight and obese women. Appetite 2010;55[3]:413–19.
10. King NA, Caudwell PP, Hopkins M, Stubbs JA, Naslund E, Blundell J. Dual process action of exercise on appetite control: increase in orexigenic drive but improvement in meal induced satiety. AJCN 2009;90[4]:921–7.
11. Boutcher SH, Dunn SL. Factors that may impede the weight loss response to exercise-based interventions. Obesity Reviews 2009;10[6]:671–80.

12. King NA, Horner K, Hills AP, Byrne NM, Wood RE, Bryant E, Caudwell P, Finlayson G, Gibbons C, Hopkins M, Martins C, Blundell JE. Exercise, appetite and weight management: understanding the compensatory responses in eating behaviour which could account for variability in exercise induced weight loss. British Journal of Sports Medicine 2011;43[12]:924–7.

13. Collins LC, Cornelius MF, Vogel RL, Walker JF, Stamford BA. Effect of caffeine and or cigarette smoking on resting energy expenditure. IJO 1994;18[8]:551–6.

14. Wing RR, Phelan S. Long term weight loss maintenance. AJCN 2005;82[1]:222S–5S.

15. Schlundt DG, Hill JO, Sbrocco T, Pope-Cordle J, Sharp T. The role of breakfast in the treatment of obesity: a randomised controlled trial. AJCN 1992;55[3]:645–51.

16. Lean ME, Lara J. Is Atkins deada (again)? Nutr Metab Cardiovasc Dis 2004;14;61–5.

17. Due A, Toubro S, Skov AR, Astrup A. Effect of normal fat diets, either medium or high in protein on body weight in overweight subjects; a randomised 1-year trial. Int J Obes 2004;28:1283–90.

18. Sullivan EL, Daniels AJ, Koegler FH, Cameron JL. Evidence in female rhesus monkeys that nightime caloric intake is not associated with weight gain. Obesity Res 2005;13:2072–80.

3 Appendices

Appendices

Appendix 1
Adult Weighing Scales
Specification Guide

All weighing equipment for use in health care settings for weighing patients for the purpose of monitoring, diagnosis and medical treatment is covered by the NAWI (Non-Automatic Weighing Instrument) regulations, and fall predominantly within Class III or Class IIII [1].

Classification of scales

Within the regulations, weighing equipment falls into four classes:

- Class I, Class II, Class III, Class IIII.

Class I scales provide the highest degree of accuracy, and Class IIII the lowest. As an example, Class IIII scales include bathroom scales for domestic use.

Recommended manufacturers and stockists usually state which class of weighing scales their products are classified as.

Scales with the capacity to weigh up to 150–250 kg should be sufficient. Scales with a higher maximum capacity will be necessary for weighing bariatric patients.

Calibration

Scales used for the weighing of patients should be regularly checked and routinely maintained to ensure correct calibration in accordance with manufacturers' instructions. Equipment should be checked regularly by standard weights (4 × 10 kg and 8 × 10 kg) and calibrated if necessary. Results of test weighing should be recorded in a book.

Reference

1. Department of Health. Medical patient weighing scales. EFA/2010/001 Estates and Facilities Alerts. http://www.dh.gov.uk/prod_consum_dh/groups/dh_digitalassets/documents/digitalasset/dh_114048.pdf; 2010.

Weight Management: A Practitioner's Guide, First Edition. Dympna Pearson and Clare Grace.
© 2012 Dympna Pearson and Clare Grace. Published 2012 by Blackwell Publishing Ltd.

Appendix 2
How to Measure Height

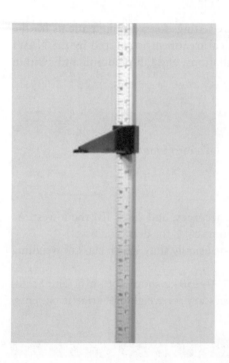

- Height is measured with a stadiometer (left).
- Patients stand in bare feet that are kept together. The head is level with a horizontal Frankfurt plane (below – an imaginary line from the lower border of the eye orbit to the auditory meatus).
- If a patient cannot stand – for example, if they are confined to a chair or bed – BMI can still be derived from equations using arm span or lower leg length instead of height.

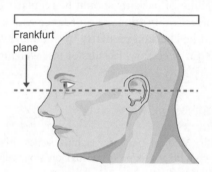

Frankfurt plane

Weight Management: A Practitioner's Guide, First Edition. Dympna Pearson and Clare Grace.
© 2012 Dympna Pearson and Clare Grace. Published 2012 by Blackwell Publishing Ltd.

Table A2.1   Height conversion table (feet/inches to metres)

ft	in	m	ft	in	m
4	0	1.22	5	3½	1.61
4	0½	1.23	5	4	1.63
4	1	1.24	5	4½	1.64
4	1½	1.26	5	5	1.65
4	2	1.27	5	5½	1.66
4	2½	1.28	5	6	1.68
4	3	1.29	5	6½	1.69
4	3½	1.31	5	7	1.70
4	4	1.32	5	7½	1.71
4	4½	1.33	5	8	1.73
4	5	1.35	5	8½	1.74
4	5½	1.36	5	9	1.75
4	6	1.37	5	9½	1.76
4	6½	1.38	5	10	1.78
4	7	1.40	5	10½	1.79
4	7½	1.41	5	11	1.80
4	8	1.42	5	11½	1.82
4	8½	1.43	6	0	1.83
4	9	1.45	6	½	1.84
4	9½	1.46	6	1	1.85
4	10	1.47	6	1½	1.87
4	10½	1.49	6	2	1.88
4	11	1.50	6	2½	1.89
4	11½	1.51	6	3	1.90
5	0	1.52	6	3½	1.92
5	0½	1.54	6	4	1.93
5	1	1.55	6	4½	1.94
5	1½	1.56	6	5	1.96
5	2	1.57	6	5½	1.97
5	2½	1.59	6	6	1.98
5	3	1.60			

Reproduced from Thomas, B. & Bishop, J. (eds) (2007) *Manual of Dietetic Practice*, 4th edn, with permission from John Wiley & Sons, Ltd.

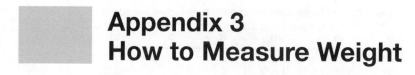

Appendix 3
How to Measure Weight

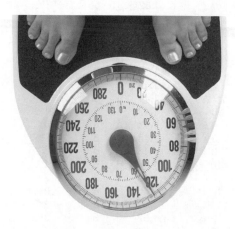

© iStockphoto.com/Julie de Leseleuc

Weight should be measured by digital scales or a beam balance to the nearest 100 g.

Measuring Weight

- Ask permission to weigh patient
- Patients should ideally be weighed in light clothing, preferably with an empty bladder
- Ask patient to remove shoes, heavy outer garments such as jackets and cardigans, heavy jewellery, loose change and keys
- Wait for scales to display 0.0 before patient stands on scales
- Ask patient to stand with their feet together in the centre and their heels against the back edge of the scales
- Arms should be hanging loosely at their sides and head facing forward. Ensure that they keep looking ahead
- Posture is important. If they stand to one side, look down, or do not otherwise have their weight evenly spread, it can affect the reading
- Provide information on weight in a neutral manner

Weight Management: A Practitioner's Guide, First Edition. Dympna Pearson and Clare Grace.
© 2012 Dympna Pearson and Clare Grace. Published 2012 by Blackwell Publishing Ltd.

Example of weighing a patient:

Practitioner: 'Are you happy for me to weight you now?'
Patient: 'If you must!'
Practitioner: 'Can I ask you to remove your shoes and jacket and any coins or keys in your pockets?'

Ensure scales is at zero before patient steps on

Practitioner: 'Make sure your feet are together, with your weight spread evenly, heels against the back of the scales. Your arms should hang loose by your sides and look straight ahead. How you stand is important, otherwise, it can affect the reading'
Practitioner: 'Would you like me to tell you what your weight is in kilograms or stones and pounds?
Patient: 'Stones and pounds. What is it?'
Practitioner: '... stones and ...pounds'. Is that what you expected?'
Patient: 'I would like it to be less, but at least it hasn't gone up!'

Table A3.1 Body weight conversion table (stones and pounds to kilograms)

st	lb	kg	st	lb	kg	st	lb	kg	st	lb	kg	st	lb	kg
0	1	0.45	6	5	40.37	9	13	63.05	13	7	85.73	17	1	108.41
	2	0.90		6	40.82	10	0	63.50		8	86.18		2	108.86
	3	1.36		7	41.28		1	63.96		9	86.64		3	109.32
	4	1.81		8	41.73		2	64.41		10	87.09		4	109.77
	5	2.27		9	42.18		3	64.86		11	87.54		5	110.22
	6	2.72		10	42.64		4	65.32		12	88.00		6	110.68
	7	3.17		11	43.09		5	65.77		13	88.45		7	111.13
	8	3.63		12	43.55		6	66.23	14	0	88.91		8	111.59
	9	4.08		13	44.00		7	66.68		1	89.36		9	112.04
	10	4.54	7	0	44.45		8	67.13		2	89.81		10	112.49
	11	4.99		1	44.91		9	67.59		3	90.27		11	112.95
	12	5.44		2	45.36		10	68.04		4	90.72		12	113.40
	13	5.90		3	45.81		11	68.49		5	91.17		13	113.85
1	0	6.35		4	46.27		12	68.95		6	91.63	18	0	114.31
2	0	12.70		5	46.72		13	69.40		7	92.08		1	114.76
3	0	19.05		6	47.17	11	0	69.85		8	92.53		2	115.21
4	0	25.40		7	47.63		1	70.31		9	92.98		3	115.67
	1	25.86		8	48.08		2	70.76		10	93.44		4	116.12
	2	26.31		9	48.54		3	71.22		11	93.90		5	116.58
	3	26.76		10	48.99		4	71.67		12	94.35		6	117.03
	4	27.22		11	49.44		5	72.12		13	94.80		7	117.48
	5	27.67		12	49.90		6	72.58	15	0	95.26		8	117.94
	6	28.12		13	50.35		7	73.03		1	95.71		9	118.39
	7	28.57	8	0	50.80		8	73.48		2	96.16		10	118.84
	8	29.03		1	51.26		9	73.94		3	96.62		11	119.30
	9	29.48		2	51.71		10	74.39		4	97.07		12	119.75
	10	29.93		3	52.16		11	74.84		5	97.52		13	120.20
	11	30.39		4	52.62		12	75.30		6	97.98	19	0	120.66
				5	53.07		13	75.75		7	98.43		1	121.11

	No.	Value		No.	Value		No.	Value		No.	Value		No.	Value
	12	30.84		6	53.52	**12**	0	76.20		8	98.88		2	121.56
	13	31.30		7	53.98		1	76.66		9	99.34		3	122.02
5	0	31.75		8	54.43		2	77.11		10	99.79		4	122.47
	1	32.21		9	54.89		3	77.57		11	100.24		5	122.93
	2	32.66		10	55.34		4	78.02		12	100.70		6	123.38
	3	33.11		11	55.79		5	78.47		13	101.15		7	123.83
	4	33.57		12	56.25		6	78.93	**16**	0	101.61		8	124.29
	5	34.02		13	56.70		7	79.38		1	102.06		9	124.74
	6	34.47	**9**	0	57.15		8	79.83		2	102.51		10	125.19
	7	34.93		1	57.61		9	80.29		3	102.97		11	125.65
	8	35.38		2	58.06		10	80.74		4	103.42		12	126.10
	9	35.83		3	58.51		11	81.19		5	103.87		13	126.55
	10	36.29		4	58.97		12	81.65		6	104.33	**20**	0	127.27
	11	36.74		5	59.42		13	82.10		7	104.79		7	130.45
	12	37.19		6	59.88	**13**	0	82.55		8	105.24	**21**	0	133.64
	13	37.65		7	60.33		1	83.01		9	105.69		7	136.82
6	0	38.10		8	60.78		2	83.46		10	106.14	**22**	0	140.00
	1	38.56		9	61.24		3	83.92		11	106.60		7	143.18
	2	39.01		10	61.69		4	84.37		12	107.04	**23**	0	146.36
	3	39.46		11	62.14		5	84.82		13	107.50	**24**	0	152.73
	4	39.92		12	62.60		6	85.28	**17**	0	107.96	**25**	0	159.09

Appendix 4
Measuring Overweight and Obesity using Body Mass Index

The National Institute for Health and Clinical Excellence (NICE) recommends that overweight and obesity are assessed using body mass index (BMI). It is used because, for most people, BMI correlates with their proportion of body fat.

BMI is defined as a person's weight in kilograms divided by their height in metres^2 (kg/m^2).

Example of how to calculate BMI

Height: 180 cm

Weight: 95 kg

BMI: $\dfrac{95\,\text{kg}}{3.24\,\text{m}^2\,(1.80 \times 1.80)} = 29\,\text{kg/m}^2$

NICE classification

Overweight	Obesity
BMI of 25–29.9 kg/m²	BMI of 30 kg/m² or more

This classification accords with that recommended by the World Health Organization (WHO).

WHO Classification of overweight/obesity in adults

Classification	BMI (kg/m²)
Healthy weight	18.5–24.9
Overweight	25–29.9
Obesity I	30–34.9
Obesity II	35–39.9
Obesity III	40 or more

These cut-off points are based on epidemiological evidence of the link between mortality and BMI in adults.

(*Source*: Department of Health. Healthy Weight, Healthy Lives: A Toolkit for Developing Local Strategies; 2008)

Weight Management: A Practitioner's Guide, First Edition. Dympna Pearson and Clare Grace.
© 2012 Dympna Pearson and Clare Grace. Published 2012 by Blackwell Publishing Ltd.

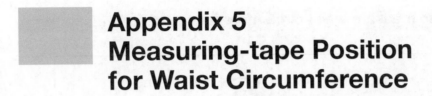

Appendix 5
Measuring-tape Position
for Waist Circumference

Measuring waist

Waist circumference is used to identify those patients with a BMI of under $35\,\text{kg/m}^2$, who may have metabolic syndrome (see Chapter 6, page 81) and therefore have significantly greater risks linked with cardiovascular disease. There is little added benefit to be gained from undertaking waist measurements for those with a BMI above $35\,\text{kg/m}^2$.

Waist measurements are more intrusive than recording weight. They need to be undertaken in a skilled and sensitive manner, with the rationale explained to the patient.

Example of discussing waist measurement

Practitioner: 'Are you happy for me to check your waist measurement?'
Patient: 'Does it make a difference?'
Practitioner: 'Yes, for some people like yourself with high blood pressure and cholesterol levels, it can be linked with a higher risk of heart problems. By checking it out, if there is a problem, it can be treated.'
Patient: 'OK, that makes sense, especially as my Dad had heart problems.'

Weight Management: A Practitioner's Guide, First Edition. Dympna Pearson and Clare Grace.
© 2012 Dympna Pearson and Clare Grace. Published 2012 by Blackwell Publishing Ltd.

How to measure waist circumference

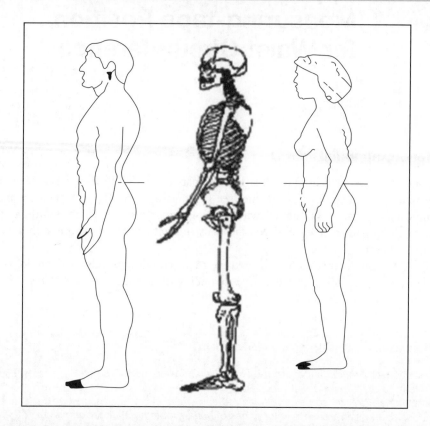

The waist circumference should be taken, with the subject standing, at the point mid-way in the mid-axillary line between the lowest rim of the rib cage and the tip of the hip bone (superior iliac crest), not at the maximum point or at the umbilicus. The measuring tape should be snug, but not so tight to the skin so as to compress it. The measurement is made at the end of a normal expiration.

(Source: National Heart, Lung and Blood Institute, "Clinical Guidelines on the Identification, Evaluation, and Treatment of Overweight and Obesity in Adults").

Appendix 6
Medications

Certain medications are known to have an adverse effect on weight and weight-management measures should be discussed with patients who are prescribed medications associated with weight gain (SIGN).

Medications known to have an adverse effect on weight

- Atypical antipsychotics, including clozapine.

- Beta adrenergic blockers, particularly propranolol.

- Insulin, when used in the treatment of type 2 diabetes mellitus.

- Lithium.

- Sodium valproate.

- Sulphonylureas, including chlorpropamide, glibenclamide, glimepiride and glipizide.

- Thiazolidinediones, including pioglitazone.

- Tricyclic antidepressants, including amitriptyline.

Weight Management: A Practitioner's Guide, First Edition. Dympna Pearson and Clare Grace.
© 2012 Dympna Pearson and Clare Grace. Published 2012 by Blackwell Publishing Ltd.

Appendix 7
Screening for
Binge-eating Disorder

Sign Guidelines [1] recommend that the following questions can be used when screening for Binge Eating Disorder (BED). If the patient answers 'yes' to all four questions, referral for specialist psychological assessment should be considered, where a more in-depth BED Questionnaire can be undertaken by a suitably qualified person.

1   Are there times during the day when you could not have stopped eating, even if you wanted to?
2   Do you ever find yourself eating unusually large amounts of food in a short period of time?
3   Do you ever feel extremely guilty or depressed afterwards?
4   Do you ever feel more determined to diet or to eat healthier after the eating episode?

(*Source*: Bruce B, Wilfley D. Binge eating among the overweight population: a serious and prevalent problem. J Am Diet Assoc 1996;96[1]:58–61.)

Reference

1.   Scottish Intercollegiate Guidelines Network. Management of Obesity: A National Clinical Guideline; 2010.

Appendix 8
General Practice Physical Activity Questionnaire

A. Calculating the 4-level physical activity index (PAI)

Patients can be classified into four categories based on the original EPIC index from which the GPPAQ was developed.

Inactive	Sedentary job and no physical exercise or cycling
Moderately inactive	Sedentary job and some but <1 hour physical exercise and/or cycling per week OR
	Standing job and no physical exercise or cycling
Moderately active	Sedentary job and 1–2.9 hours physical exercise and/or cycling per week OR
	Standing job and some but <1 hour physical exercise and/or cycling per week OR
	Physical job and no physical exercise or cycling
Active	Sedentary job and ≥3 hours physical exercise and/or cycling per week OR
	Standing job and 1–2.9 hours physical exercise and/or cycling per week OR
	Physical job and some but <1 hour physical exercise and/or cycling per week OR
	Heavy manual job

Note: Questions concerning Walking, Housework/Childcare and Gardening/DIY have been included to allow patients to record their physical activity in these categories, however these questions have not been shown to yield data of a sufficient reliability to contribute to an understanding of overall physical activity levels. As noted above further questioning is required.

B. Summary of the PAI

Physical exercise and/or cycling (hr/wk)	Occupation			
	Sedentary	Standing	Physical	Heavy Manual
0	Inactive	Moderately Inactive	Moderately Active	Active
Some but <1	Moderately Inactive	Moderately Active	Active	Active
1–2.9	Moderately Active	Active	Active	Active
≥3	Active	Active	Active	Active

Date_____

Name_____

NHS

1. Please tell us the type and amount of physical activity involved in your work.

		Please mark one box only
a	I am not in employment (e.g. retired, retired for health reasons, unemployed, fulltime carer etc.)	
b	I spend most of my time at work sitting (such as in an office)	
c	I spend most of my time at work standing or walking. However, my work does not require much intense physical effort (e.g. shop assistant, hairdresser, security guard, childminder, etc.)	
d	My work involves definite physical effort including handling of heavy objects and use of tools (e.g. plumber, electrician, carpenter, cleaner, hospital nurse, gardener, postal delivery workers etc.)	
e	My work involves vigorous physical activity including handling of very heavy object (e.g. scaffolder, construction worker, refuse collector, etc.)	

2. During the *last week*, how many hours did you spend on each of the following activities? *Please answer whether you are in employment or not*

Please mark one box only on each row

		None	Some but less than 1 hour	1 hour but less than 3 hours	3 hours or more
a	Physical exercise such as swimming, jogging, aerobics, football, tennis, gym workout etc.				
b	Cycling, including cycling to work and during leisure time				
c	Walking, including walking to work, shopping, for pleasure etc.				
d	Housework/Childcare				
e	Gardening/DIY				

3. How would you describe your usual walking pace? Please mark one box only.

Slow pace (i.e. less than 3 mph) [ ]   Steady average pace [ ]

Brisk pace [ ]   Fast pace (i.e. over 4mph) [ ]

Appendix 9

PAR-Q & YOU

Physical Activity Readiness
Questionnaire - PAR-Q
(revised 2002)

(A Questionnaire for People Aged 15 to 69)

Regular physical activity is fun and healthy, and increasingly more people are starting to become more active every day. Being more active is very safe for most people. However, some people should check with their doctor before they start becoming much more physically active.

If you are planning to become much more physically active than you are now, start by answering the seven questions in the box below. If you are between the ages of 15 and 69, the PAR-Q will tell you if you should check with your doctor before you start. If you are over 69 years of age, and you are not used to being very active, check with your doctor.

Common sense is your best guide when you answer these questions. Please read the questions carefully and answer each one honestly: check YES or NO.

YES	NO	
☐	☐	1. Has your doctor ever said that you have a heart condition <u>and</u> that you should only do physical activity recommended by a doctor?
☐	☐	2. Do you feel pain in your chest when you do physical activity?
☐	☐	3. In the past month, have you had chest pain when you were not doing physical activity?
☐	☐	4. Do you lose your balance because of dizziness or do you ever lose consciousness?
☐	☐	5. Do you have a bone or joint problem (for example, back, knee or hip) that could be made worse by a change in your physical activity?
☐	☐	6. Is your doctor currently prescribing drugs (for example, water pills) for your blood pressure or heart condition?
☐	☐	7. Do you know of <u>any other reason</u> why you should not do physical activity?

Weight Management: A Practitioner's Guide, First Edition. Dympna Pearson and Clare Grace.
© 2012 Dympna Pearson and Clare Grace. Published 2012 by Blackwell Publishing Ltd.

If you answered

YES to one or more questions

Talk with your doctor by phone or in person BEFORE you start becoming much more physically active or BEFORE you have a fitness appraisal. Tell your doctor about the PAR-Q and which questions you answered YES.

- You may be able to do any activity you want — as long as you start slowly and build up gradually. Or, you may need to restrict your activities to those which are safe for you. Talk with your doctor about the kinds of activities you wish to participate in and follow his/her advice.
- Find out which community programs are safe and helpful for you.

NO to all questions

If you answered NO honestly to all PAR-Q questions, you can be reasonably sure that you can:

- start becoming much more physically active — begin slowly and build up gradually. This is the safest and easiest way to go.
- take part in a fitness appraisal — this is an excellent way to determine your basic fitness so that you can plan the best way for you to live actively. It is also highly recommended that you have your blood pressure evaluated. If your reading is over 144/94, talk with your doctor before you start becoming much more physically active.

DELAY BECOMING MUCH MORE ACTIVE:

- if you are not feeling well because of a temporary illness such as a cold or a fever — wait until you feel better; or
- if you are or may be pregnant — talk to your doctor before you start becoming more active.

PLEASE NOTE: If your health changes so that you then answer YES to any of the above questions, tell your fitness or health professional. Ask whether you should change your physical activity plan.

Informed Use of the PAR-Q: The Canadian Society for Exercise Physiology, Health Canada, and their agents assume no liability for persons who undertake physical activity, and if in doubt after completing this questionnaire, consult your doctor prior to physical activity.

No changes permitted. You are encouraged to photocopy the PAR-Q but only if you use the entire form.

NOTE: If the PAR-Q is being given to a person before he or she participates in a physical activity program or a fitness appraisal, this section may be used for legal or administrative purposes.

"I have read, understood and completed this questionnaire. Any questions I had were answered to my full satisfaction."

NAME _____

SIGNATURE _____ DATE _____

SIGNATURE OF PARENT _____ WITNESS _____
or GUARDIAN (for participants under the age of majority)

Note: This physical activity clearance is valid for a maximum of 12 months from the date it is completed and becomes invalid if your condition changes so that you would answer YES to any of the seven questions.

© Canadian Society for Exercise Physiology www.csep.ca/forms

CSEP | SCPE
THE GOLD STANDARD IN EXERCISE
SCIENCE AND PROFESSIONAL TRAINING

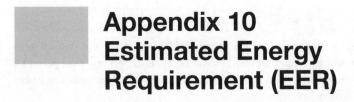

Appendix 10
Estimated Energy
Requirement (EER)

Daily estimated energy requirements to maintain body weight are calculated using a formula to account for four factors: gender, age, activity level and current weight. Modest energy-deficit diets, which would achieve about 0.5 kg (1 lb) a week weight loss, are based on daily dietary intake of 600 calories less than the person's daily energy requirement. Work out the patient's 'Estimated energy requirements for a 600-calorie energy-deficit diet' using the information below. This information uses the Schofield and WHO energy-requirement equations, but we recognise that there are alternative equations that you may prefer to use.

BMR

Based on the patient's age, gender and current weight (in kg) as listed in the chart below, predict their Basal Metabolic Rate (BMR). This is based on modified Schofield equations (see the Department of Health's Dietary Reference Values, 1991).

Age range for men and women

Basal metabolic rate equals:

Age	Men	Women
18–29 years	15.1 × weight (kg) + 692	14.8 × weight (kg) + 487
30–59 years	11.5 × weight (kg) + 873	8.3 × weight (kg) + 846
60+ years	11.9 × weight (kg) + 700	9.2 × weight (kg) + 687

Weight Management: A Practitioner's Guide, First Edition. Dympna Pearson and Clare Grace.
© 2012 Dympna Pearson and Clare Grace. Published 2012 by Blackwell Publishing Ltd.

PAL

Incorporate the patient's Physical Activity Level (PAL) based on the gender and activity levels shown in the chart below. Do this by multiplying the patient's estimated BMR with the appropriate figure from the table. Few patients are likely to have activity levels above 'inactive'.

Activity level	Description	Men	Women
Inactive	Assume sitting most of the day with less than 2 hours on their feet.	**1.4**	**1.4**
Light	Assume some daily exercise – at work or tasks about the house or garden – with at least 2 hours on their feet.	**1.5**	**1.5**
Moderate	Assume 6 hours on their feet or regular strenuous exercise.	**1.78**	**1.64**
Heavy	Those in heavy labouring jobs or serious athletes in training.	**2.1**	**1.82**

EER

Calculate the patient's daily estimated energy requirement to maintain weight by multiplying BMR and PAL.

EER for weight loss

Subtract 600 calories from the above figure to estimate the patient's energy requirement for modest weight loss.

(*Source*: DOM UK/NDRI.)

Appendix 11
Prescribed Energy Deficit
(PED)-Ready Reckoner

Female

18–30 years

Wt (kg)	Wt (stone)	Inactive	Light	Mod	Heavy
60–70	9'6–11'1	1200	1500	1500	2000
71–75	11'2–11'12	1500	1800	2000	2300
76–80	11'13–12'9	1500	2000	2000	2300
81–85	12'10–13'6	1500	2000	2000	2500
86–90	13'7–14'3	1500	2000	2300	2500
91–100	14'4–15'11	1800	2300	2500	2500
101–114	15'12–18'0	2000	2500	2500	2500
115–125	18'1–19'10	2300	2500	2500	2500
>125	19'10	2500	2500	2500	2500

31–60 years

Wt (kg)	Wt (stone)	Inactive	Light	Mod	Heavy
60–70	9'6–11'1	1200	1500	1500	1800
71–75	11'2–11'12	1200	1500	1800	2000
76–80	11'13–12"9	1200	1800	1800	2000
81–95	12'10–15'0	1500	1800	2000	2300
96–114	15'1–18'0	1500	2000	2300	2500
115–130	18'1–20'7	1800	2300	2300	2500
131–150	20'8–23'9	2000	2500	2500	2500
151–170	23'10–26'12	2300	2500	2500	2500
>170	>26'12	2500	2500	2500	2500

Weight Management: A Practitioner's Guide, First Edition. Dympna Pearson and Clare Grace.
© 2012 Dympna Pearson and Clare Grace. Published 2012 by Blackwell Publishing Ltd.

Over 60 years

Wt (kg)	Wt (stone)	Inactive	Light	Mod	Heavy
60–65	9'6–10'5	1200	1200	1500	1500
66–75	10'6–11'12	1200	1500	1500	1800
76–85	11'13–13'6	1200	1500	1800	2000
86–95	13'7–15'0	1500	1800	2000	2000
96–100	15'1–15'11	1500	2000	2000	2300
101–110	15'12–17'5	1500	2000	2000	2500
111–120	17'6–18'13	1500	2000	2300	2500
121–135	19'0–21'4	1800	2300	2500	2500
136–165	21'5–26'1	2000	2500	2500	2500
>165	>26'1	2500	2500	2500	2500

Male

18–30 years

Wt (kg)	Wt (stone)	Inactive	Light	Mod	Heavy
60–65	9'6–10'5	1500	1800	2300	2800
66–70	10'6–11'1	1500	2000	2500	3000
71–75	11'2–11'12	1500	2000	2500	3000
76–80	11'13–12'9	1800	2300	2500	3000
81–85	12'10–13'6	1800	2300	2800	3000
86–95	13'7–15'0	2000	2500	3000	3000
96–110	15'1–17'5	2300	2800	3000	3000
111–125	17'6–19'10	2500	3000	3000	3000
126–135	19'11–21'4	2800	3000	3000	3000
>135	>21'4	3000	3000	3000	3000

31–60 years

Wt (kg)	Wt (stone)	Inactive	Light	Mod	Heavy
60–75	9'6–10'5	1500	1800	2300	2800
66–70	10'6–11'1	1500	2000	2300	2800
71–75	11'2–11'12	1500	2000	2500	3000
76–80	11'13–12'9	1800	2000	2500	3000
81–85	12'10–13'6	1800	2300	2500	3000
86–90	13'7–14'3	1800	2300	2800	3000
91–110	14'4–17'5	2000	2500	2800	3000
111–120	17'6–18'13	2300	2800	3000	3000
121–150	19'0–23'9	2500	3000	3000	3000
151–160	23'10–25'4	2800	3000	3000	3000
>160	>25'4	3000	3000	3000	3000

Over 60 years

Wt (kg)	Wt (stone)	Inactive	Light	Mod	Heavy
60–65	9'6–10'5	1200	1500	1800	2000
66–70	10'6–11'1	1200	1500	1800	2300
71–75	11'2–11'12	1200	1500	2000	2500
76–80	11'13–12'9	1500	1800	2000	2500
81–85	12'10–13'6	1500	1800	2300	2800
86–95	13'7–15'0	1500	2000	2300	2800
96–100	15'1–15'11	1800	2000	2500	3000
101–110	15'12–17'5	1800	2300	2800	3000
111–125	17'6–19'10	2000	2500	3000	3000
126–135	19'11–21'4	2300	2800	3000	3000
136–165	21'5–26'1	2500	3000	3000	3000
>165	>26'1	3000	3000	3000	3000

Light Activity: Some daily activity (at work or tasks about the house or garden) with at least 2 hours on their feet.
Moderate Activity: Assumes 6 hours on their feet or regular strenuous activity.
Heavy: Those in heavy labouring jobs or serious athletes in training.

Appendix 12
Portions Commonly Used for the 'Eatwell Plate' (To Check Nutritional Adequacy of the Diet)

Household measures: 1 portion of:

Cooked vegetables or salad	= cricket ball
Fruit	= 1 handful
Boiled potato	= 1 egg
Baked potato	= computer mouse
Cooked rice, pasta	= tennis ball
Meat, poultry	= deck of cards
Fish	= chequebook
Jams or dressings	= golf ball
Cheese	= matchbox

Table A12.1 What is a portion? (TBS = tablespoon)

Food group	A portion
Fruit & vegetables	3 TBS cooked vegetables 1 small cereal bowl salad 1 medium tomato 1 small corn on the cob 1 glass fruit juice (100 ml) 1 medium apple, banana, orange Small bunch grapes (10–12) 1 large slice of melon 3 TBS tinned fruit 3 dried apricots 1 TBS raisins, sultanas

(*continued*)

Weight Management: A Practitioner's Guide, First Edition. Dympna Pearson and Clare Grace.
© 2012 Dympna Pearson and Clare Grace. Published 2012 by Blackwell Publishing Ltd.

Table A12.1   *(cont'd)*

Food group	A portion
Bread, cereals, rice, potato, pasta	3 TBS breakfast cereal 2 TBS muesli 3 TBS porridge oats 1 weetabix or shredded wheat 1 slice bread/toast ½ large roll ½ pitta bread 1 small chappati 2 crispbreads or crackers 2 TBS boiled rice (1 oz uncooked) 3 TBS cooked pasta (1 oz uncooked) 2 egg-sized potatoes (100 g = 4 ozs) 2 TBS mashed potato 8 oven chips 1 crumpet/pancake 1 small slice of malt loaf ½ scone or ½ English muffin
Dairy foods	⅓ pint milk (200 ml) 1 yogurt (125 g/5 oz pot) 1 oz (25 g) hard cheese 2 oz (50 g) low fat cheese 5 oz. (125 g) pot cottage cheese
Protein foods	2–3 ozs (60–90 g) meat/poultry 5 ozs (125 g) fish 2 eggs 4–5 TBS baked beans, chick peas, pulses 2 TBS (40 g) nuts 4 ozs (120 g) Quorn/tofu/soya
Fats	1 teaspoon of butter/margarine/oil 2 teaspoons of ½ butter/margarine 1 teaspoon mayonnaise/cream
Extras = 50 kcals	1 fruit 1 plain biscuit 1 Jaffa cake/fig roll 1 scoop plain ice cream 1 low calorie soup/hot chocolate 2 teaspoons jam 1 pub measure of spirits
Extras = 100 kcals	1 fun size chocolate bar 1 chocolate digestive/hobnob 2 plain biscuits 1 low fat bag crisps ½ pint cider ½ pint beer 1 small glass wine
Extras = 150 kcals	1 packet crisps 1 chocolate covered biscuit 1 choc ice 1 chocolate biscuit 1 oz peanuts 5 TBS Bombay mix 1 large glass wine 1 pint beer

Appendix 13
Example of 1500 kcal based on 'Eatwell Plate' Portions

Time	Food	Carbohydrate	Fruit and Vegetables	Dairy	Protein	Fat	Extras
8.00 am	Mug of tea (350 ml) with 40 ml of semi-skimmed milk						
8.15 am	2 medium slices of wholemeal bread toast (36 g each), 1 teaspoon of butter (7 g)	2				1	
9.00 am	Mug of coffee (350 ml) with 40 ml of semi-skimmed milk						
10.00 am	Mug of coffee (350 ml) with 40 ml of semi-skimmed milk and low-fat fruit yoghurt (110 g)			1			
12.30 am	2 medium slices of white bread (36 g each), 1 tablespoon of light mayonnaise (20 g), 1 large egg (50 g) and fruit juice drink (250 ml carton)	2	2		0.5	1	

(continued)

Weight Management: A Practitioner's Guide, First Edition. Dympna Pearson and Clare Grace.
© 2012 Dympna Pearson and Clare Grace. Published 2012 by Blackwell Publishing Ltd.

Time	Food	Carbohydrate	Fruit and Vegetables	Dairy	Protein	Fat	Extras
3.00 pm	Mug of coffee (350 ml) with 40 ml of semi-skimmed milk and 1 gingernut biscuit						45
5.00 pm	1 apple (88 g)		1				
7.00 pm	1 × 140 g skinless chicken breast roasted, 200 g of frozen vegetables boiled, 215 g of new potatoes boiled with skin	2	2		1.5		
8.00 pm	65 g of green grapes, 19 g of mature cheddar cheese and 1 small glass of red wine (125 ml)		1	1			85
	Semi-skimmed milk in tea: 200 ml (⅓ of a pint)			1			
	Totals	**6**	**6**	**3**	**2**	**2**	**130 kcal**

Appendix 14
Example of 1800 kcal based on 'Eatwell Plate' Portions

Time	Food	Carbohydrate	Fruit and vegetables	Dairy	Protein	Fat	Extras
8.00 am	Mug of tea (350 ml) with 40 ml of semi-skimmed milk						
8.15 am	2 medium-cut slices of wholemeal bread toasted (36 g each), 2 teaspoon of butter (14 g), 2 tablespoons of jam	2				2	50
9.00 am	Mug of coffee (350 ml) with 40 ml of semi-skimmed milk						
10.00 am	Mug of coffee (350 ml) with 40 ml of semi skimmed milk and low-fat fruit yogurt (110 g)			1			
12.30 am	2 medium-cut slices of white bread (36 g each), 1 tablespoon of light mayonnaise (20 g), 1 large egg (50 g) and fruit juice drink (250 ml carton)	2	2		0.5	1	

(continued)

Weight Management: A Practitioner's Guide, First Edition. Dympna Pearson and Clare Grace.
© 2012 Dympna Pearson and Clare Grace. Published 2012 by Blackwell Publishing Ltd.

Time	Food	Carbohydrate	Fruit and vegetables	Dairy	Protein	Fat	Extras
3.00 pm	Mug of coffee (350 ml) with 40 ml of semi-skimmed milk and a gingernut biscuit (10 g)						45
5.00 pm	1 apple (88 g)		1				
7.00 pm	1 × 140 g of skinless chicken breast roasted, 200 g of frozen vegetables boiled, 215 g new potatoes boiled with skin	2	2		1.5		
8.00 pm	4 rye crackers (40 g), 130 g of green grapes, 19 g of mature cheddar cheese and 1 small glass of red wine (125 ml)	2	2	1			85
	Semi-skimmed milk in tea: 200 ml (⅓ of a pint)			1			
	Totals	**8**	**7**	**3**	**2**	**3**	**180 kcal**

Appendix 15
Cookery Books

1. Good Housekeeping. Light & Healthy Cooking: 250 Delicious, Satisfying, Guilt-Free Recipes. Hearst Books. 2012.
2. Hornby J. Good Food: 101 Healthy Eats: Triple-tested Recipes. BBC Books; 2008.
3. Humphries C. The Classic 1000 Calorie-counted Recipes. W Foulsham & Co Ltd; 1998.
4. Good Food: Low-fat Feasts: Triple-tested Recipes (BBC Good Food). 2003.
5. Good Food: 101 Healthy Eats – Triple tested recipes (BBC Good Food). 2008.
6. The Essential Low Fat Cookbook (in association with HEART UK). Anthony Worral Thompson. 2011.
7. Weight Watchers New Complete Cookbook. Wiley Publishing, 2010.
8. Weight Watchers Simply the Best: 250 Prizewinning Family Recipes. Weight Watchers Publishing Group. 1997.
9. Healthy meal, healthy hearts [South Asian free recipe book]. British Heart Foundation (www.bhf.org.uk/publications).
10. The Biggest Loser Cookbook – your personal programme for nutritious and delicious guilt free food – Hamlyn. 2012.

Weight Management: A Practitioner's Guide, First Edition. Dympna Pearson and Clare Grace.
© 2012 Dympna Pearson and Clare Grace. Published 2012 by Blackwell Publishing Ltd.

Appendix 16
NICE Guidance on Referral to Slimming Groups

NICE recommends that primary care and local authorities recommend self-help, commercial and community weight-management programmes only if they follow best practice, as defined by programmes which:

- Help people assess their weight and decide on a realistic healthy target weight loss (usually 5–10%).
- Aim for maximum weekly weight losses of 0.5–1 kg.
- Focus on long-term lifestyle changes rather than short-term, quick-fix approaches.
- Are multicomponent, addressing diet and activity and offering a variety of approaches.
- Use a balanced, healthy eating approach.
- Recommend regular physical activity (particularly activities that can be part of daily life, such as brisk walking and gardening) and offer practical, safe advice about being more active.
- Include some behaviour-change techniques, such as keeping a diary, and advice on how to cope with 'lapses' and 'high-risk' situations.
- Recommend and/or provide ongoing support.

Weight Management: A Practitioner's Guide, First Edition. Dympna Pearson and Clare Grace.
© 2012 Dympna Pearson and Clare Grace. Published 2012 by Blackwell Publishing Ltd.

Appendix 17
Weighed Portions for Where More Precision is Required

Food group	A weighed portion
Fruit and vegetables Calorie content per portion = 40 kcal	1 fruit, e.g. 85 g apple, 65 g orange, 40 g banana Large helping vegetables, e.g. 170 g carrot 60 g peas, 170 g broccoli, 250 g cabbage 1 large salad, 330 g 1 small glass fruit juice, 110 ml
Bread, cereals, rice, potato, pasta Calorie content per portion = 80 kcal	3 dspn Cereal, e.g. 25 g branflakes or cornflakes 1 slice wholemeal bread, 40 g 3 dspn rice, 60 g 3 dspn cooked pasta, 50 g (or 80 g spaghetti) 2 small potatoes (100 g)
Dairy Calorie content per portion = 90 kcal	265 ml semi-skimmed milk 1 yogurt, 115 g pot Cheddar cheese, 22 g
Protein Calorie content per portion = 140 kcal	75 g pork chop, 65 g salmon, 150 g cod 2 eggs, 95 g 4 dsps baked beans, 170 g
Fats Calorie content per portion = 50 kcal	5 g fat = 1 tsp butter/margarine/oil
Examples of extras	50 kcal = 1 fruit, 1 plain biscuit 100 kcal = 125 ml glass wine, 50 g ice cream 150 kcal = 1 packet crisps, 1 chocolate biscuit, 2 small glasses wine

tsp = teaspoon, dspn = dessertspoon.

Why are these portion sizes different from those used in Appendix 12?

Portion sizes used in Appendix 12 are based on household measures and many people can successfully lose weight using household measures as a guide for portion sizes. However, when weight loss does not happen, more precision is required on actual weighed amounts. It is recommended that these portion sizes are used when more precision is required for a carefully calorie-controlled diet. These are based on the detailed portion sizes provided in Resource 26.

Weight Management: A Practitioner's Guide, First Edition. Dympna Pearson and Clare Grace.
© 2012 Dympna Pearson and Clare Grace. Published 2012 by Blackwell Publishing Ltd.

4 Resources

List of Resources

1. Implicit Association Test – self assessment of attitudes, https://implicit.harvard.edu/implicit/demo/index.jsp.
2. Bias Educational videos, www.yaleruddcenter.org.
3. DOMUK Position Paper on Very Low Energy Diets, www.domuk.org.
4. Department of Health. Thinking of Having a Baby: Folic Acid – An Essential Ingredient in Making Babies. http://www.food.gov.uk/multimedia/pdfs/publication/thinkingbaby0908.pdf.
5. Department of Health. The Pregnancy Book. http://www.ndr-uk.org/downloads/pdf/weightmgt/MaternalWeightManagement/110117Maternal%20weight%20management%20PIL.pdf.
6. Change4Life, http://www.nhs.uk/change4life/Pages/change-for-life.aspx.
7. Cancer Research UK. Ten Top Tips for a Healthy Weight – Based on Scientific Evidence. Order from: http://publications.cancerresearchuk.org.
8. Department of Health. Why Weight Matters. Order from: http://www.dh.gov.uk/en/Publicationsandstatistics/Publications/index.htm.
9. Department of Health. Your Weight, Your Health. Order from: http://www.dh.gov.uk/en/Publicationsandstatistics/Publications/PublicationsPolicyAndGuidance/DH_4134408.
10. Video for measuring height: NHANES III anthropometric procedure videos, http://www.cdc.gov/nchs/video/nhanes3_anthropometry/height/height.htm.
11. Video of measuring weight: NHANES III anthropometric procedure videos, http://www.cdc.gov/nchs/video/nhanes3_anthropometry/weight/weight.htm.
12. Video of measuring waist: NHANES III anthropometric procedure videos, http://www.cdc.gov/nchs/video/nhanes3_anthropometry/circumference/circumference.htm.
13. Willson R, Veale D, Clarke A. Overcoming Body Image Problems. Robinson; 2009.
14. Cash TF. The Body Image Workbook: An 8-Step Program for Learning to Like Your Looks. Oakland, CA: New Harbinger Publications; 1997.
15. Fairburn CG. Overcoming Binge Eating. The Guilford Press; 1995.
16. The Healthy Portion Plate, healthyportionplate.com.

17   Carbs & Cals, http://www.carbsandcals.com/About.aspx.
18   Weight Loss Resources: Calorie Carb and Fat Bible 2011, http://www.weightlossresources.co.uk/lostart.htm.
19   Collins UK. Collins Gem - Calorie Counter. Collins UK; 2013.
20   Humphries C. Pocket Calorie Counter: The Little Book That Measures and Counts Your Portions Too. Foulsham; 2008.
21   Weight Loss Resources: Food & Exercise Daily Diary, http://www.weightlossresources.co.uk/shop/weight-loss-products/food-exercise-diary.htm.
22   Gauntlett-Gilbert J, Grace C. Overcoming Weight Problems. Robinson; 2005.
23   Humphries C. The Classic 1000 Calorie-counted Recipes. Foulsham; 1998.
24   NHS Choices: food labels, http://www.nhs.uk/Livewell/Goodfood/Pages/food-labelling.aspx.
25   NHS Choices: The 'eatwell plate', http://www.nhs.uk/Livewell/Goodfood/Pages/eatwell-plate.aspx.
26   Nutrition and Diet Resources UK, http://www.ndr-uk.org/.
27   British Heart Foundation. 1) Take Control of Your Weight. 2) So You Want to Lose Weight. Both available from http://www.bhf.org.uk/publications/publications-search-results.aspx?m=simple&q=weight.

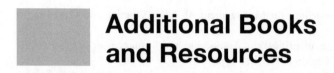

Additional Books and Resources

Books

Costain L. Diet Trials: How to Succeed at Dieting. BBC Publication; 2003.
Gauntlett-Gilbert J, Grace C. Overcoming Weight Problems. Robinson; 2005.
Kopleman P. Management of Obesity and Related Disorders. Martin Dunitz; 2001.
Kushner RF, Bessessen DH. Evaluation & Management of Obesity. Hanley & Belfus; 2001.
Wadden TA, Stunkard AJ. Handbook of Obesity Treatment. Guilford Press; 2004.

Useful Web sites

ASO (Association for Study of Obesity), www.aso.org.uk.
BDA (British Dietetic Association), www.bda.uk.com.
BHF (British Heart Foundation), www.bhf.org.uk.
BNF (British Nutrition Foundation), www.nutrition.org.uk.
Department of Health: Obesity, http://www.dh.gov.uk/en/Publichealth/Obesity/index.htm.
National Obesity Observatory, www.noo.org.uk.
National Weight Control Registry, www.nwcr.ws.
NICE (National Institute of Clinical Excellence), www.nice.org.uk.
NIH (National Institute of Health, USA): Obesity, http://www.nhlbi.nih.gov/guidelines/
    obesity/ob_home.htm.
NOF (National Obesity Forum), www.nationalobesityforum.org.
SIGN (Scottish Intercollegiate Guidelines Network), www.sign.ac.uk.
Weight Concern, www.weightconcern.com.

Guidelines and Reports

Department of Health, Healthy Weight, Healthy Lives: A Toolkit for Developing Local Strategies.
    http://www.dh.gov.uk/en/Publicationsandstatistics/Publications/DH_088968; 2008.
Health Survey for England, http://www.ic.nhs.uk/statistics-and-data-collections/health-and-
    lifestyles-related-surveys/health-survey-for-england.
National Audit Office. Tackling Obesity in England. National Audit Office; 2001. The
    Stationery Office. Report by the Controller and Auditor General. London: The Stationery
    Office. www.nao.gov.uk.

Weight Management: A Practitioner's Guide, First Edition. Dympna Pearson and Clare Grace.
© 2012 Dympna Pearson and Clare Grace. Published 2012 by Blackwell Publishing Ltd.

National Obesity Forum. Guidelines on Management of Adult Obesity and Overweight. NOF; 2001.

NICE. Obesity: The Prevention, Identification, Assessment and Management of Overweight and Obesity in Adults and Children. NICE; 2006.

Scottish Intercollegiate Guidelines Network. Obesity: A National Clinical Guideline for Use in Scotland. Edinburgh: SIGN; 2010.

Tackling Obesities: The Foresight Report. http://www.idea.gov.uk/idk/core/page.do?pageld=8267926; 2007.

WHO. Obesity: Preventing and Managing the Global Epidemic: Report of the World Health Organization Consultation on Obesity. Geneva: World Health Organization; 2000.

5 Tools

Tool 1
Weight History Chart

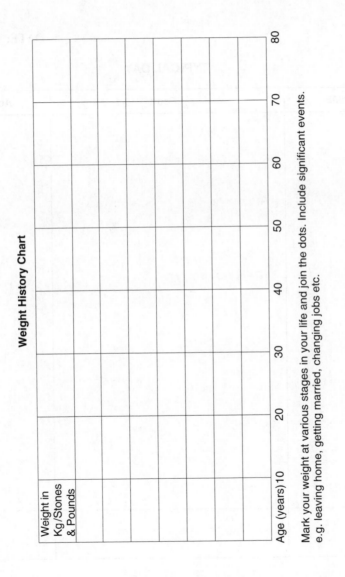

Weight History Chart

Weight in Kg/Stones & Pounds

Age (years) 10   20   30   40   50   60   70   80

Mark your weight at various stages in your life and join the dots. Include significant events. e.g. leaving home, getting married, changing jobs etc.

Weight Management: A Practitioner's Guide, First Edition. Dympna Pearson and Clare Grace.
© 2012 Dympna Pearson and Clare Grace. Published 2012 by Blackwell Publishing Ltd.

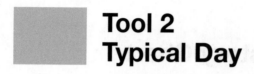

Tool 2
Typical Day

DATE:

TYPICAL DAY

TIME	Food	Activity

Tool 3
Activity Charts

24 hours

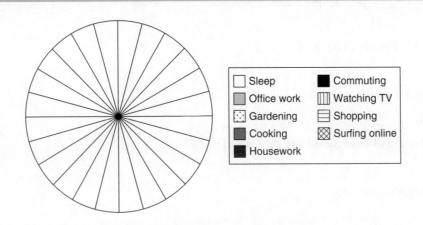

Sleep	Commuting
Office work	Watching TV
Gardening	Shopping
Cooking	Surfing online
Housework	

Time spent on activity (minutes)

TIME	ACTIVITY	Time (minutes)

Steps recorded

Mon	Tue	Wed	Thu	Fri	Sat	Sun

Weight Management: A Practitioner's Guide, First Edition. Dympna Pearson and Clare Grace.
© 2012 Dympna Pearson and Clare Grace. Published 2012 by Blackwell Publishing Ltd.

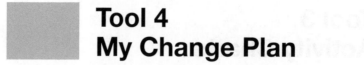

Tool 4
My Change Plan

What change do I intend to make?

What needs to be in place?

What might get in the way?

How will I get round any difficulties?

Who might help?

Do I need to talk to them?

When will I start?

How will I check if I am doing it?

Anything that might help me keep it up (rewards)?

Date to review progress:

Tool 5
Plate Model

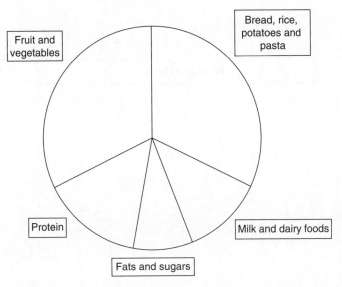

Fruit and vegetables

Bread, rice, potatoes and pasta

Protein

Milk and dairy foods

Fats and sugars

Put a tick (√) in each section for foods consumed from each of the food groups and compare to the 'eatwell plate'.

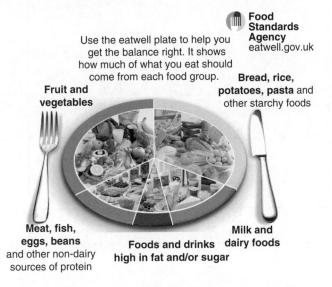

Use the eatwell plate to help you get the balance right. It shows how much of what you eat should come from each food group.

Food Standards Agency
eatwell.gov.uk

Fruit and vegetables

Bread, rice, potatoes, pasta and other starchy foods

Meat, fish, eggs, beans and other non-dairy sources of protein

Foods and drinks high in fat and/or sugar

Milk and dairy foods

Weight Management: A Practitioner's Guide, First Edition. Dympna Pearson and Clare Grace.
© 2012 Dympna Pearson and Clare Grace. Published 2012 by Blackwell Publishing Ltd.

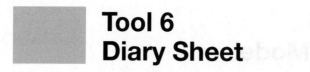

Tool 6
Diary Sheet

Time	Food and Drink	Activity

Weight Management: A Practitioner's Guide, First Edition. Dympna Pearson and Clare Grace.
© 2012 Dympna Pearson and Clare Grace. Published 2012 by Blackwell Publishing Ltd.

Tool 7
Weight Record Chart

Kg Pounds	WEIGHT	Week 1	Week 2	Week 3	Week 4	Week 5	Week 6	Week 7	Week 8	Week 9	Week 10	Week 11	Week 12
Start													
–1													
–2													
–3													
–4													
–5													
–6													
–7													
–8													
–8													
–8													
–9													
–10													
–11													
–12													
–13													
–14													
–15													
–16													
–17													
–18													
–19													
–20													

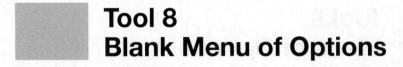

Tool 8
Blank Menu of Options

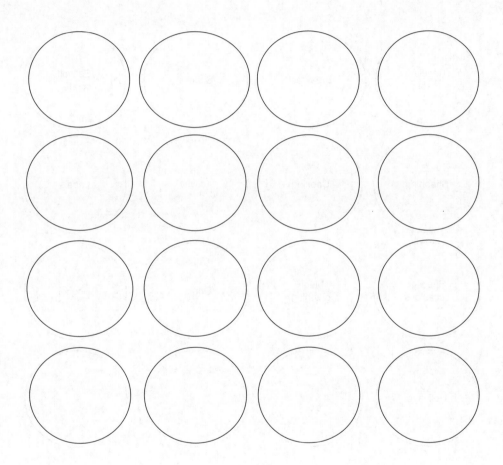

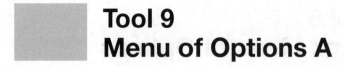

Tool 9
Menu of Options A

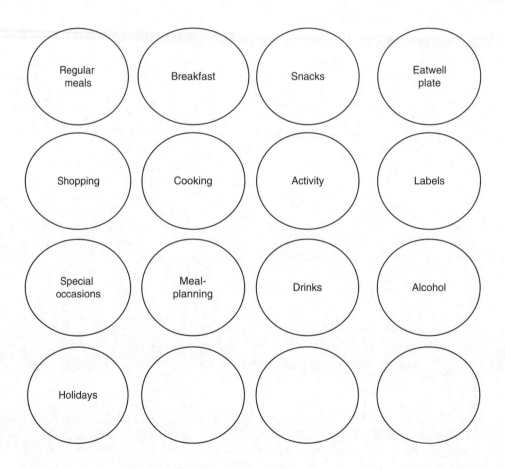

Regular meals	Breakfast	Snacks	Eatwell plate
Shopping	Cooking	Activity	Labels
Special occasions	Meal-planning	Drinks	Alcohol
Holidays			

Tool 10
Menu of Options B

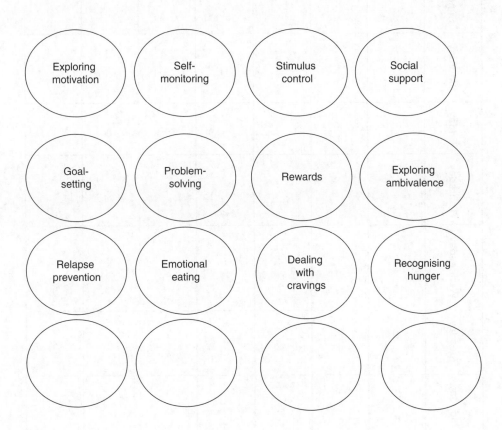

Exploring motivation	Self-monitoring	Stimulus control	Social support
Goal-setting	Problem-solving	Rewards	Exploring ambivalence
Relapse prevention	Emotional eating	Dealing with cravings	Recognising hunger

Weight Management: A Practitioner's Guide, First Edition. Dympna Pearson and Clare Grace.
© 2012 Dympna Pearson and Clare Grace. Published 2012 by Blackwell Publishing Ltd.

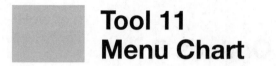

Tool 11
Menu Chart

TIME	Monday	Tuesday	Wednesday	Thursday	Friday	Saturday	Sunday
Breakfast							
Mid-morning							
Lunch							
Afternoon							
Evening							
Milk for drinks							
Extras							

Weight Management: A Practitioner's Guide, First Edition. Dympna Pearson and Clare Grace.
© 2012 Dympna Pearson and Clare Grace. Published 2012 by Blackwell Publishing Ltd.

Tool 12
Assessment of Diet Quality

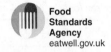

Food
Standards
Agency
eatwell.gov.uk

Use the eatwell plate to help you get the balance right. It shows how
much of what you eat should come from each food group.

**Fruit and
vegetables**

**Bread, rice,
potatoes, pasta**
and other starchy foods

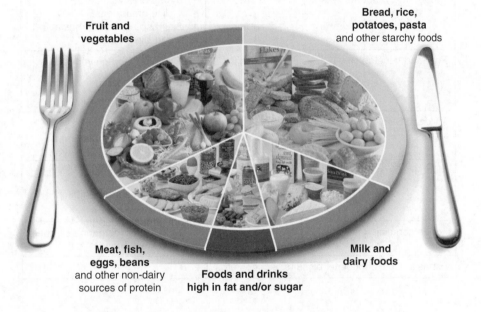

**Meat, fish,
eggs, beans**
and other non-dairy
sources of protein

**Foods and drinks
high in fat and/or sugar**

**Milk and
dairy foods**

(Eatwell plate reproduced courtesy of Department of Health (2011).)

Daily Portions based on The Eat Well Plate

Food Group	1500 kcals	1800 kcals	Your Portions
Bread, rice, potatoes, pasta	6	8	
Fruit and vegetables	6	7	
Milk and dairy foods	3	3	
Meat, fish, eggs, beans	2	2	
Foods containing fat	2	3	
Extras (crisps, chocolate, biscuits, alcohol, etc.)	130 kcals	180 kcals	

Food Group	What Counts as a Portion
Bread, rice, potatoes, pasta	<ul><li>3 tbsp breakfast cereal</li><li>1 slice bread/toast</li><li>2–3 tbsp boiled rice/pasta</li><li>2 egg size potatoes</li></ul>
Fruit and Vegetables	<ul><li>1 medium portion vegetables</li><li>Salad</li><li>1 medium fruit</li><li>1 small glass fruit juice</li></ul>
Milk and Dairy Foods	<ul><li>1 glass milk (⅓ pint)</li><li>1 pot yogurt</li><li>1 matchbox piece cheese</li></ul>
Meat, fish, eggs, beans	<ul><li>2–3 oz cooked meat</li><li>5 oz fish</li><li>2 eggs</li><li>5 tbs baked beans</li></ul>
Foods containing fat	<ul><li>1 tsp butter/margarine/oil/ghee</li><li>1 tsp mayonnaise</li></ul>
Extras (crisps, chocolate, biscuits, alcohol, etc.)	

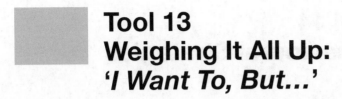

Tool 13
Weighing It All Up:
'I Want To, But...'

	Advantages	Disadvantages
C H A N G E	*What are the good things about making changes to my eating and activity?*	*What are the not-so-good things about making changes to my eating and activity?*
N O C H A N G E	*What would be good about not having to change my eating or activity?*	*What would be the not-so-good things about not changing my eating or activity?*

Weight Management: A Practitioner's Guide, First Edition. Dympna Pearson and Clare Grace.
© 2012 Dympna Pearson and Clare Grace. Published 2012 by Blackwell Publishing Ltd.

Tool 14
Behavioural Strategies

- ☐ Do nothing else whilst eating; focus and sit down at a table.
- ☐ Don't eat when watching TV or reading.
- ☐ Have a glass of water with your meal.
- ☐ Spend longer eating meals.
- ☐ Savour your food – eat slowly and enjoy each mouthful.
- ☐ Chew each mouthful thoroughly, 10–20 times.
- ☐ Cut food into smaller, bite-sized pieces.
- ☐ Put your knife and fork down between mouthfuls.
- ☐ Use cutlery rather than your fingers.
- ☐ Use a smaller plate or bowl.
- ☐ Put food away – out of sight.
- ☐ Always shop from a list.
- ☐ Never shop on an empty stomach.
- ☐ Keep busy and on the move.
- ☐ Break up sedentary activities like watching TV into short episodes.
- ☐ Don't sit for longer than half an hour.
- ☐ Plan menus for the week ahead.
- ☐ Plan activity for the week ahead.
- ☐ Put leftovers in the freezer.
- ☐ Clean your teeth after a meal.

Weight Management: A Practitioner's Guide, First Edition. Dympna Pearson and Clare Grace.
© 2012 Dympna Pearson and Clare Grace. Published 2012 by Blackwell Publishing Ltd.

Index

Note: Page numbers in *italics* refer to Figures; those in **bold** to Tables.

Weight Management: A Practitioner's Guide, First Edition. Dympna Pearson and Clare Grace.
© 2012 Dympna Pearson and Clare Grace. Published 2012 by Blackwell Publishing Ltd.